Community Care in England and France

Reforms and the improvement of equity and efficiency

BLEDDYN DAVIES
JOSÉ FERNÁNDEZ
ROBIN SAUNDERS

Routledge
Taylor & Francis Group
LONDON AND NEW YORK

First published 1998 by Ashgate Publishing

Reissued 2018 by Routledge
2 Park Square, Milton Park, Abingdon, Oxon, OX14 4RN
711 Third Avenue, New York, NY 10017, USA

Routledge is an imprint of the Taylor & Francis Group, an informa business

A Library of Congress record exists under LC control number: 98071404

Typeset by Jane Dennett at the PSSRU, University of Kent at Canterbury

ISBN 13: 978-1-138-62449-8 (hbk)
ISBN 13: 978-0-429-46076-0 (ebk)

Contents

Part II

Part III

List of tables, boxes and figures

Tables

Boxes

Figures

Preface by Marie-Jo Guisset

The idea of a comparative overview of the French and English systems of domiciliary care for elderly people had its roots in the visits to Kent by French gerontological teams.[1] It finally saw the light of day in 1992.

La Fondation de France had several reasons for financing this study in Athis Mons, La Manche and St Omer. At one level, it reflected the increasing awareness in France of care management and a desire to learn more, following its widespread introduction in England and Wales after April 1993 as a result of the National Health Service and Community Care Act 1990. At another level, it contributed to the intense and long-lasting debate over nearly ten years, over the allowance for dependent elderly people, which has just been formalised in the PSD (*prestation spécifique dépendance*).

It seemed worthwhile, therefore, to compare how the systems worked in Great Britain and in France in terms of: those systems which allocate resources for the care at home of dependent elderly people; their effects on the demand for entry into residential care; and the role of the informal sector in the provision of care for the elderly. These represent a whole range of highly topical questions for each of our two countries.

Despite the adversity of our legislation and the complexity of the financing system in France, the research team from the PSSRU has managed to produce an extremely interesting comparative analysis. It illuminates the choices faced by the funding agencies and the work of those at local level, so that the new view of ageing which *la Fondation de France* is seeking to develop will come to be reflected in the intentions of legislators and everyday reality.

Mme Marie-Jo Guisset
Responsable des Actions Personnes Agées
Fondation de France

1 Study visits organised by *INRAC Grand Age* (*Institut national pour la retraite active*, Paris) in conjunction with PSSRU, University of Kent.

Introduction

Study foci

Foci and research questions. This book is about equity and efficiency in England and France. After giving an account of institutions and of the history of development and reform in the two countries, it summarises the results of a comparative empirical study of aspects of equity in care consumption and efficiency in care production. Another book, produced with a grant from the British Council, will contain a more detailed description of English and French policy and institutions and an analysis of the literatures about equity and efficiency.

The equity and efficiency concerns determined the research question: who obtains *how much* help with the *activities of daily living* from *what source,* at what *costs of public funds,* and with *what effects*?

By *who,* we mean 'what persons with what need-related characteristics'. By *how much,* we mean the number of hours of assistance. By the *activities of daily living,* we mean tasks of everyday life such as personal care and supervision (e.g. washing, grooming, feeding), and household care (e.g. the procurement of adequately attractive and nutritrious meals, transfer to and from bed, keeping the home warm and tidy, shopping), and related tasks like help with administrative activities. By *source,* we mean persons from the family and other parts of the *entourage* who are not paid a sum of money for the tasks on the basis of a formal contract, or various organisations for whom a major goal is the provision of services in response to difficulties with precisely such tasks. By *costs to public funds,* we mean financing from a collective source financed by compulsory contributions, including taxation.

The two countries have complex policy aims. However, both have adopted what the OECD has claimed to be the highest common factor of reform goals among all the countries investing in reform: to provide choice to a higher proportion of persons at high risk of unwanted entry to institutions for long-term care (OECD, 1994). That is the main *effect* measured in this study.

Why the study?

We undertook these Anglo-French comparisons for two reasons. First, France and England[2] are here sufficiently in common for contrasts to be stimulating. They are among the longest established of the main European states, as well as the closest of neighbours. Unsurprisingly, therefore, they have a degree of similarity which makes contrast interesting. For two thousand years, they have been societies at more broadly similar stages of development than one would have thought from older textbooks of European history. They have similar per capita incomes. They share common values. There is much in common between France and Great Britain in the 'technology' used by organisations to care for elderly people: for instance, the *maison de retraite* corresponds broadly to the elderly persons' home, and *aide ménagère* corresponds broadly to the home help service. There are similarities also in broad values, expectations and beliefs applied by citizens' families and by policy-makers. Both countries have developed publicly-subsidised services since the war to much the same levels of provision. (Within Europe, contrast England and France with Greece and Portugal; OECD, 1996, chapter 2.) Both acknowledge a public responsibility for minimum care provisions and standards. In both societies, individuals value their autonomy and privacy more greatly than in China, for instance (Olson, 1993). Without these similarities, the contrasts would stretch our imaginations much less productively. In their different ways, both France and Great Britain are currently engaged in the reform of community and long-term care. It is therefore natural for both to look to the outside world, both to compare the equity and efficiency of their policy efforts and also, by explaining differences, to gain insights into how to make their own systems better.

But their interdependence makes their analysis still more interesting. At the time of writing, the European Union seems to be the Millennium Dome of international alliances: a structure of great political symbolism under which there will surely be important activity of as yet an unpredictable kind. In no century of this millennium have England and France failed to have powerful impacts on one another. Arguably, they are one of a group of nations which have almost established their sense of identity by their contrasts. But the signs are that their interdependence

2 For England, read England and Wales, the study including Welsh data.

will be still greater in the next millennium. The degree of competition between producers from economies within the frontiers of the Union will surely increase. In many of the sectors which will make the running, the important players in the new economies will not be truly national at all. It is a cliché of our times that once economies are opened, the capacity of the governments of nation states to dominate becomes progressively less. The pressures of the Europe-wide economic competition will increasingly shape all policy. And it is difficult to see how the European economy can insulate itself from an increasingly competitive world economy and so drive towards improved efficiency. That will put new constraints on social policy. Indeed, it will create what Richard Titmuss feared: a social policy whose values themselves more closely reflect the values of economic policy, in one sense more in the mainstream tradition of some European welfare states, but in another, profoundly different from them in its emphasis on efficiency in the production of welfare.

Throughout the post-war world, the British have become progressively more aware of the limitations of an open economy in a competitive world on their domestic policies. The French have become aware of this only more recently. Among the effects is a determination among many in France to know more about other societies. This is reflected in more widespread reading of English language literatures. That it might be of use to some French as well as British readers also encouraged us to do the study.

Study design. The British evidence is from a study of 589 new elderly recipients of community social services in England and Wales, during the period immediately prior to the reform heralded by the National Health Service and Community Care Act of 1990. The persons were drawn from twelve small areas in ten local authorities. The French evidence is a study of 198 new elderly recipients of the comparable services for which data were collected between 1992 and 1994 in three areas. The data relate to three points in time: assessment, six months and twelve months later. The French study aimed to collect data comparable to the most essential of the data collected in the earlier British study.

Book contents

The book has three broad parts.

Part I is primarily an analytic description of institutions and policy ideas. Readers who know one system well are unlikely to know as much about the other. So we considered this analytic description to be necessary in order to set the context of the empirical study, and outline the study design.

Chapter 1 opens with an analytic account of the differences between the two systems. It describes how there are important ways in which political authority, responsibility and accountability are more defined and concentrated in the UK; how there is a different balance between subsidy in cash and kind; how, in France, eligibility criteria are focused more on the individual and disability, less on the handicapped people in the broader social and material context which influence the need judgements of British agencies. However, it shows that with respect to the principal 'outcome' of this study of needs, resources and outcomes, the levels of utilisation of residential institutions are broadly similar. That is so although the conceptualisation of equity and efficiency are as different in focus and (in some respects) stage of development as are the factors which influence the actual degrees of equity and efficiency by the criteria of each country.

Chapter 2 is about home care in England. It discusses pre-reform provision, particularly access and assessment; development of the intellectual basis and practical content of the reforms during each of three periods since the mid-seventies. It also discusses its post-reform characteristics around propositions about the implications of the consolidation of institutional functions and the clarity with which issues are defined, the new dominance of independent providers, and the introduction of a care management process and system, the new mechanism for securing equity and efficiency at the level of the individual.

Chapter 3 first describes the development of the principal French services, again discussing access, assessment structures and the incentives which they create. It reviews the French critique of the system, illustrating how similar are many of the criticisms to those of the pre-reform British system. Then it describes the logic, content and consequences of successive reform attempts. The study of these attempts illuminates the nature of French institutions and processes. It also illustrates how the timing of attempts at reform in a narrow policy area are affected by broad national and international pressures. It discusses the degree to which the reforms put in place help to provide a framework for improving equity and efficiency.

Part II is about the empirical study. Chapter 4 describes its design. Evidence was collected for three sites in France, and compared with evidence for three sites in England and Wales, the sites being broadly matched for socio-economic characteristics.

The three French sites contrasted with respect to their delivery models. One gave a priority to the payment of cash allowances to finance care rather than to service provision. A second had a unified nursing and home help service. A third had separate services but provided a single point of entry to home nursing, home help and *garde à domicile.* The sites were Athis Mons (a suburb of Paris), La Manche (a *département* of Normandy), and St Omer and its hinterland (a light industrial and market town in the Pas de Calais).

The information collected in France included dependency characteristics, the structure of the household and the family, housing circumstances and social contacts, other data about needs, whether the user was eligible for public subsidy through *aide sociale,* the hours of service requested and agreed or the cash equivalent, hours of input of informal help for care tasks, and service utilisation, including admissions to institutions. Full data were collected for the time of assessment and six months later for both countries, and it was possible to compare the probabilities of admission to residential institutions after twelve months.

Chapter 5 compares the need-related circumstances of the samples of beneficiaries in each of the three pairs of areas.

Chapter 6 presents the analyses of service utilisation. A main theme is the substitution (that is, replacement) in the French areas of formal for informal care for individuals as the case history unfolds. The analysis is based partly on a path model relating individual circumstances to informal care, and formal provision and changes in them over the three points of time. The analysis is based also on an extension of an approach pioneered by Tennstedt et al. (1993). The authors had extended the analytic framework by allowing also for substitution across tasks as well as overall. But they had restricted their analysis to the investigation of *whether* there was substitution, not estimating the *amount* of substitution. This analysis extends the approach by estimating the amount of substitution, and the degree to which this was likely to have reflected justifiable relief of unacceptable caregiver stress and other circumstances. It found that there was little replacement which might be due to other than increasing needs or unacceptable stress on caregivers. The results are compatible with most of the findings from the albeit cruder studies in Anglo-Saxon countries.[3] That no such effect was evident in France by the mid-nineties suggests that it is not an imminent danger there. Perhaps its emergence is inhibited by the existence of the *obligation alimentaire*, the wide household and family obligation to accept financial responsibility for provision to elderly persons.

Chapter 7 analyses the probability of admission to institutions for long-term care. On the one hand, the study finds the British system to be more effective in making admission to institutions unnecessary over the period of the study for individually matched samples, the probability for English users being approximately one-half that for French users. On the other, it finds that the marginal productivity of the French cash benefit *allocation compensatrice pour tierce personne* with respect to admission to institutions is much higher than that of its English counterpart. It also finds low marginal productivities for service inputs in both countries.

There is an appendix table which provides some additional analyses from the collection. It is included because there does not seem to be other French evidence of quite the same kind.

Part III is an overview of the results and argument. Chapter 8 first summarises the main findings about the need-related circumstances of users, the help received from informal caregivers, the use of formal agency services, and the probability of admission to institutions for long-term care. Then, it discusses what light the findings throw on the key differences between the two systems, and whether the reforms in the two countries provide a better foundation for long-run improvements in equity and efficiency. Its arguments encourage optimism about what might be achieved with continued policy investment in the long run in both countries, although it is only fair to admit that the futures are to differing degrees uncertain, and that many in both countries would be less optimistic about what opportunities the reforms present.

3 However, the study for one cohort of individuals over a short period of time is unable to refute the argument that, over a substantial period of time, there could be such a substitution effect.

Acknowledgments

The work was financed and enabled by *la Fondation de France*. Through its project officer, Mlle Marie-Jo Guisset, the Fondation found areas willing to participate, did much to negotiate the provision of the information to us, and provided the home for meetings in Paris with the collaborating teams from the three areas. The project could not have taken place without dynamism and networking skills. Indeed, Mlle Guisset was one of the true originators of the project, perhaps its main originator. With Mme Nicolle Lépine, Mlle Guisset had been involved in the management of twice-yearly visits by parties of senior French care professionals and managers to the University of Kent, the visits having taken place over a period of more than a decade. The visitors had talks from PSSRU staff based on Unit work and the British social services in general, and paid visits of observation from their Kent base. Those visits established networks which were later to be drawn on in this project. Indeed, they are one source of the knowledge of British argument and innovations which French policy-makers and analysts have increasingly brought to bear on their own work in various parts of France, and the critiques of their system in some of the state documents of the late eighties and early nineties. Some of the connections will be seen by the careful reader of this book.

We are indebted also to those from the collaborating French agencies. They supervised the collection of the data. Through their membership of the steering committee, they participated in guiding the design of the collection, analysis and interpretation of data. We returned from our visits recharged with their enthusiasm and captivated by their hospitality. They were of enormous help in interpreting as well as collecting the evidence, although they cannot be held responsible for imperfections in the design and conduct of the research and the argument created from it. Among those who contributed most were Professor Michel Frossard who provided costs data, and Mme Scholl of Levallois-Perret (92) who provided detailed costs on institutional care and other technical material. We are grateful to M. Boudreau, *Direction de l'action social* of the *Caisse national d'assurance vieillesse* (75), M. Robinne of Coutances (50) and M. Vignon (75) for insights into the functioning of the funding of domiciliary care, including the newer forms of service provision. Mme Nicole Lépine of the *Institut national pour la retraite active* (75) and Professors Jean-Claude Henrard and Alain Grand, collaborators in another project on Franco-British policy development in community and long-term care of elderly people, have in various ways helped and influenced our argument. Finally, there are those who contributed to the analysis and production of the report at the University of Kent: Barry Baines, Steve Carter and Peter Ely who contributed academic assistance; and Audrey Walker, Jane Dennett and Nick Brawn whose arduous work made the report ready for publication. We trust that all those who have helped will find what we have produced interesting and useful.

We are also grateful to Ashgate, who have handled the book with characteristic professionalism.

Part I

1 English and French policy goals and service systems: vivent les différences

Arrangements for securing the financing and provision of services reflect the different broad models of social policy of which each is an example: often (inadequately) described as Bismarckian social insurance model supplemented with social assistance in France; the 'Beveridgean welfare state' model in England. Esping-Andersen (1990) described characteristics of the social insurance model as 'conservative' and 'corporatist'. French commentators themselves have identified these characteristics in the French system (Henrard, 1994).

Each of a number of differences between the English and French systems can be hypothesised to affect many aspects of the efficiency of the systems.

1. Concentration of responsibility, authority and accountability

It could be expected that the greater the concentration of responsibility, authority and accountability for setting and achieving goals, the greater its efficiency. The less the concentration, it might be hypothesised, the more difficult would be coordinated policy action at all levels, reflecting the greater diffusion of power and so the greater number of conflicting goals to be reconciled;[1] and the less likely would be the flexibility in the distribution and use of resources through time required for achieving important and changing goals effectively and efficiently.

The British system has inherited a high degree of concentration of authority, responsibility and accountability at every level: the political and national executive level, the local level, and the field level. In the

1 A report from the Commissariat général du plan on the health services and their financing commented: *'Là où nous pêchons, c'est par l'application .... Sans doute, est-ce là une constante du mal français: l'idée tient parfois lieu d'action'* (Soubie et al., 1994, p.228).

French system, they are fragmented at all of these levels, as is commonly found in countries with variants of a Bismarckian social insurance model.

The financing system is considered to be complex and rigid (Joel and Martin, 1994). The *caisses de retraite* are particularly important because they have a discretionary role in financing home care of the *aide ménagère* (home help) type. They were separated from the *assurances maladie* only in 1967 (Henrard et al., 1991, p.101). The financial position of the *caisses* differs greatly, reflecting the fortunes of industries and occupational groups and, in particular, the ratios of beneficiaries (retired people) to contributors (in paid employment). They have had great latitude in their policies for the subsidisation of home help. Therefore, the *caisses* operate different policies about what level of subsidy for home care is given to whom (Curtis et al., 1992; Commissariat général du plan, 1991, p.55; Henrard, 1994).[2]

The structure of the system can make it difficult for the *caisses* to implement a targeting policy. The outcome of CNAV Circulaire No. 86/93 is an example. Issued by the national director of CNAV (Caisse nationale d'assurance vieillesse), it was intended to improve targeting of home help provision on the most dependent, by requiring each region to attain a quota whereby 6 per cent of cases would receive over 30 hours help per month. The regions were reluctant to accept this, since it was often at variance with their own targeting criteria. So also were service providers. However, in their case, this was because in many *départements*, the *conseils généraux* had a separate policy of favouring payment of the ACTP cash allowance to dependent elderly people. The effect of that was to debar the recipients from receiving intensive levels of home help, thus frustrating the service provider's efforts to meet the CNAV 6 per cent quota.

At the regional, county and larger municipality levels, there is again diversity in responsibility, authority and accountability for financing. For example, within the framework of the *régime géneral*, the *assurance*

2 The white paper on the funding of health services produced an overwhelming list of arguments in favour of the unification of *assurances maladie* (Soubie et al., 1994). The *assurances vieillesse* are more varied. That may make the unification of their benefits more difficult, since the habit has been to assume that the state will bail out the weaker organisations, and allow the strong to resist the loss of the privileges gained by their beneficiaries.

maladie (CNAM) has regional tiers of *conseils d'administration* who jealously guard their autonomy in the implementation of the national policy.

This fragmentation of financing affects supply, so working through to the level of the small area and the individual case. The criticisms include some made in the UK since the late seventies. There are many examples.

• People tend not to choose to enter homes, and do not play an active part in the processes by which they end up there: *'il est en effet remarquable que l'initiative d'entrée en établissement échappe presque entièrement à l'intéressé'* (Attias-Donfut et al., 1994, p.20).

• *Aide ménagère* is not particularly targeted at those with great handicap.[3]

• The tasks performed are neither those which correspond to the handicaps of the recipients,[4] nor the ones which make admission to

---

3 *'... ce qui indique bien que la prestation n'est pas ciblée sur la dépendance'* (Joel and Martin, 1994, p.138), repeating the same inference in the Schopflin report (Commissariat général du plan, 1991, p.55). Earlier, Attias-Donfut and Rozenkier (1981) had shown that 57 per cent of cases suffered little or no disability. Guillemard and Frossard (1993, p.259) quote a study suggesting both that 35 per cent of recipients of *aide ménagère* do not need it, and that 21 per cent of requests are not satisfied. During the same period, Colvez et al. (1985), defining targeting priorities around the availability and provision of informal care and disability and handicap, estimated vertical target efficiency to be approximately 60 per cent. Applying the set definitions of target groups and definitions of vertical target efficiency used in Bebbington and Davies (1983) to the same database as used by Colvez and his colleagues, Curtis estimated that by no targeting criterion did the degree of vertical target efficiency exceed 67 per cent in Ile de France, though that, she estimated, was much higher than for London and the Home Counties (Curtis, 1986).

4 *'Il est à noter que, bien souvent, les aides ménagères effectuent les tâches que les personnes âgées peuvent accomplir sans difficulté'* (Henrard and Ankri, 1994, p.112). Also, *'En effet, cette prestation ne présente ni la technicité soignante que peut eventuellement requérir l'état de la personne âgée dépendante ni la plasticité d'emploi que lui permettrait d'asssurer une présence de grande amplitude et une aide à l'accomplissement des actes essentiels de la vie courante, même si dans la pratique, des aides ménagères se prêtent à de telles interventions.'* ... *'Dans l'étàt actuel des choses, l'aide ménagère apparait comme une prestation indispensable au fonctionnement du maintien à domicile, mais dont l'orientation vers le soutien aux plus dépendants apparait impraticable sans réforme profonde du système'* (Commissariat général du plan, 1991, pp.55, 57).

institutions for long-term care most likely. For instance, they provide too little sitting for the relief of carers, and there is insufficient flexibility in the timing of interventions: it is not available out of office hours, at weekends and on bank holidays, for example.

• Instead of reforming the existing services and consolidating them into coherent structures at the local level, with the concentration of authority and responsibility and accountability for their coordination, services 'have been piled on top of one another without any general arrangement for making them coherent' (Guillemard and Frossard, 1993, p.256). Henrard (1994) likewise writes of a system of innovation by *'sédimentation'*.[5]

• Assessment practice has varied greatly. One consequence is that some progressive organisations have been attempting to make the outcomes of the assessment process more reliable by the use of standardised assessment forms and reviewing allocations as needs change (Curtis et al., 1992, p.350; Colvez et al., 1995; Puech and Colvez, 1995). Another is that there has been pressure to standardise the assessment protocols used in allocating the new benefit (*'prestation'*) for long-term care for elderly people. There is the same interest in second-generation assessment-focused systems of the RAI (resident assessment instrument) type among some French research groups as there is in other countries.

However, there are problems which are different. For instance, the *médecins libéraux* (fee-for-service general practitioners) are an all-affecting source of distortion, particularly when associated with the high prestige and great power of the medical profession. There are more physicians in relation to the population than in England, and they compete for patients in the fee-for-service system. They therefore have an incentive not to gate-keep like the British GP.[6]

---

5 The CNAV's more flexible and tightly targeted service supplementing *aide ménagère* discussed below in the text had precisely the characteristics aimed at for all non-routine practical care in current British policy, judging from the description (Gouriou, 1993).

6 Immediately prior to the mid-1997 elections, the Juppé government were attempting two changes which would affect the consequences of the activities of the *médecins libéraux* for community and long-term care. One, proposed by CNAM but rejected by many of the medical unions, would, among other things, introduce sanctions against doctors who did not complete the new *carnet de santé*, also known as the *dossier unique*. This would provide a single

The consciousness of ineffectiveness and fragmentation is one reason for the French preoccupation with coordination since the Lion report of 1981 (Commissariat général du plan, 1981). The Schopflin report perceived coordination to be one of the three preconditions for efficiency/effectiveness (*'efficacité'*) of the home care services (Commissariat général du plan, 1991, p.54).[7,8] The logic of the demonstration projects launched by Simone Weil and supported by President Chirac combines the *prestation dépendance*[9] with care management features: a

---

record of all medical services received by each patient, somewhat similar to the existing system of a patient's medical records as in the UK (*Actualités sociales hebdomadaire*, no. 1996, 8 November 1996). The other proposed reform was to reduce by five thousand the number of *médecins libéraux* by such measures as early retirement, in order to reduce the number of prescribers, with the expectation that this would thus reduce the number of medicines prescribed (*Le Monde*, 24 April 1997). Concurrently, it was proposed to introduce experimental *filières et réseaux de soins*, which would constrain direct access to specialists (*Actualités sociales hebdomadaire*, no. 1989, 20 September 1996). The long series of strikes by doctors in training just prior to the calling of the general election reflects the strength of the deeply entrenched opposition within the medical profession. The current system receives support from the public because there is a distrust of British-style waiting lists and rationing on the one hand, and the gross inequalities of access and care in the American system, on the other.

7 The distinction is made between coordination at the agency level, and co-ordination *'au niveau de la terre'*. Some argument about the care management role implies the targeting of the later stages of care management mainly at those without families, who under subsidiarity and the *obligation alimentaire* with *solidarité entre les générations*, are assumed to play whatever of those care management tasks are needed themselves: *'Lorsque la famille ne peut jouer son rôle normal, un référent unique est nécessaire pour une même personne, qu'elle soit à domicile ou en établissement'* (Commissariat général du plan, 1991, p.52).

8 Echoing some analysts in the UK and the US during the seventies and eighties, some perceive the marginal productivity of additional service inputs to be lower than the marginal productivity of care management: *'de manière très rapide, d'importants moyens collectifs ont été mis en place, bien que parfois encore en dessous du souhaitable. C'est l'efficacité de cet ensemble qui doit être améliorée dans la prochaine décennie'* (Commissariat général du plan, 1991, p.54). Compare Piktialis (1981) about the State of Massachusetts in the seventies and eighties.

9 The form of the benefit in the experiments is in cash, is not chargeable to

standardised assessment protocol, a coordination around the person and family to provide the information and *'son orientation pour leur utilisation'*; and coordination of the packaging of service.

The *'dualisme'* between health and social care of which the French complain exists in the UK also, save that the metaphor suggests sets of almost irreconcilable bipolarities and oppositions. And in the UK, the structural separation and cultural, procedural and institutional differences were, until recently at any rate, accompanied by a larger community care system covering a higher proportion of long-term care; one whose role is being extended by the more systematic redistribution of the community and long-term care function from health to social care. The effect is to concentrate long-term care in community social care which has itself been made more coherent.

An economically (or fiscally) efficient choice between modes of care is less likely in France. One reason is that the English concept, 'value for money', has not been consistently promoted by leaders of French policy opinion for the choice of care mode, despite some small studies in the late eighties and one distinguished work published in the early nineties (Bouget et al., 1990). In contrast, the economics of the costs and benefits of individual choices of alternative care models has been an important and well-published theme of the policy-analytic critiques which preceded the English reforms of the early nineties (Audit Commission, 1985, 1986; Davies and Challis, 1986; Davies et al., 1990).

A second reason is the fragmentation of the system in France. The British system has an arrangement which creates pressure for the benefits and costs to the public funders of individuals' choice of care mode to be taken into account. For instance, authorities are increasingly encouraging care managers to take into account costs to the social services department. In contrast, although the French system has as one of its aims the support of persons at home, and its critiques comment on the excessive propensity to enter institutions, there are few arrangements to make the system efficient in that respect, or even to make the professional workers conscious of the need to do so.

---

the family or to the estate after death, and is not taxable (*Le Monde*, 20 May 1994, p.22).

2. Balance between benefits in cash and kind

The guiding metaphor in France being insurance, the subsidy is seen as an entitlement, if claimants demonstrate the 'insured event'. Cash benefits have played a larger part than in the UK: *'dans le système français, il s'agit surtout de prestations en espèces ou d'aides fiscales et exonérations sociales. Les services et prestations en nature occupent une place marginale'* (Commissariat général du plan, 1991). Attendance allowance is the principal cash benefit to users for the procurement of care in the UK. The nearest French equivalent is the *allocation compensatrice pour tierce personnes* (ACTP).[10]

Since 1987, fiscal subsidies and the simplification of procedures in France have raised the incentives to use the ACTP to employ help directly. There has been continuous publicity which has raised its profile — including, most recently, widespread political justification of the benefits by their effects on generating employment. Its flexibility has been praised (Commissariat général du plan, 1991). The effect is to create competition between direct employment and the consumption of formal services.[11]

Figure 1 compares the English levels measured thus with the distribution in the French data. It will be seen how much higher the cash benefit can be in France in proportion to the relevant cost of residential care. However, in neither does there appear to be a clear correlation between the probability of receiving the benefits and the level of disability, save that in France the ACTP is not received by the least disabled.

---

10 The *caisses de retraite*, particularly CNAV, used their funds to support *aide ménagère* from the early seventies, the public assistance authorities doing the same in the eighties (Schopflin, 1991, p.51). The *allocation compensatrice* was introduced with legislation in 1975.

11 Writing about the ACTP, it has been argued that, taken with generating direct employment, an important aim in French policy, it has *'de très grands avantages de souplesse. Ses possibilitiés de modulation permettent de tenir compte du degré de handicap. Sa qualité de prestation en espèce évite la professionalisation systématique du soutien à domicile et encourage à la personnne âgée dépendante à faire appel à son entourage et à sa famille'* (Commissariat général du plan, 1991, p.58). So, far from there being a fear of paying the family, such payments are seen as promoting *solidarité*. Chirac has made employment generation a general criterion for the evaluation of all policies.

Figure 1. Attendance allowance (AA) and ACTP: amounts received as percentage of national residential care cost and proportions of recipients by disability range

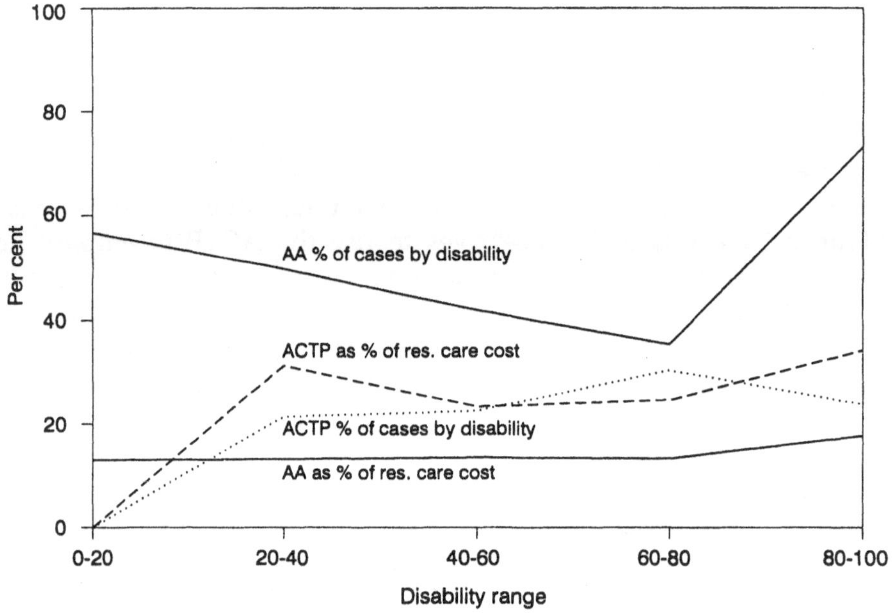

3. Focus of eligibility on the person

In France, this too follows from the application of the insurance metaphor. The focus of eligibility is the individual.

However, there is considerable gerontological evidence showing how the incidence of subsidies is substantially determined by the provision of informal caregiving in most countries, irrespective of financing system. Applying eligibility and allocation criteria based solely on dependence causes either those in most need according to the judgements to obtain too little on average, or programme costs to be much increased (Davies, 1992). The argument has been particularly important in Israel and the USA (Habib and Windmiller, 1992). It is partly for this reason that, despite the difficulties in defining objectives (Capitman, 1994), the discussion of eligibility and allocation criteria has shifted to concepts like the three discussed by Spector and Kemper (1994): the total hours of help needed; the hours of needs currently unmet after taking into account the informal care input; and the total hours of need with care plans based on needs unmet after an acceptable contribution from informal caregivers.

The French express concern about the excessive focus on the individual in determining eligibility.[12] The French distortion is also recognised in the Schopflin report.[13] That is one reason why, in 1992, only 160,000 received ACTP while there were more than 500,000 persons who were heavily dependent (Henrard and Ankri, 1994, p.120).

4. Proportions living in residential institutions and receiving home care

American literature on the nursing home market clearly shows the influence of the supply of places in institutions for long-term care on the probability of entry, irrespective of the provision of home care services. It is difficult to make precise statistical comparisons between the two countries. The OECD reported that the proportions of elderly persons in residential homes were almost identical in 1990: 5.0 per cent in France, and 5.1 per cent in the UK (OECD, 1996, Table 3.1). The report placed France and the UK in the same group with respect to the proportions in institutions (Figure 3.1). However, as late as 1980, when the social security system began to finance rapidly increasing

---

12 *'Il y a une conception très individualiste de la protection sociale. On aide des individus isolés, indépendamment de leur contexte. Cette conception a un avantage: les personnes sont autonomisées. Mais ce n'est pas toujours le cas'* (Attias-Donfut et al., 1994, p.19). The Schopflin report saw the capacity to sustain, mobilise, inform and in part to train the social support system, recognising their anxieties and needs, as another of the three preconditions for effective/efficient home care (Commissariat général du plan, 1991, p.54).

13 *'Les soins produits par l'entourage complètent une production professionelle de soins oú s'y substituent partiellement. ... l'importance de la production domestique de soins aux personnes âgées est généralement sous-estimée, voire ignorée'* (Commissariat général du plan, 1991, p.60).

proportions in British residential care, the proportions were lower in France. Curtis (1986, Table 4) compared population census data, finding that although for persons aged 85 and over the proportions living in institutions for long-term care were similar, the rates were 65 per cent greater in France for the younger elderly aged under 75 years, and 36 per cent greater for those aged between 75 and 85.

The French competitive economy of supply of residential care is without powerful mechanisms to maximise the ratio of benefits to costs to public funds for individual cases in the selection of care at home. The supply level was substantially driven by the financing mechanism, itself substantially the product of the workings of the broad social insurance model. In contrast, rates of utilisation of home care are higher in the UK. A comparison of French provision in 1984/5 with English provision in 1991 suggested that the proportions of the younger elderly receiving *aide ménagère* and *soins à domicile* were not greatly different in the two countries, though the proportion of those aged 75 and over using home help was higher in the UK (Henrard, 1992, Table 24).

On three of these four counts, the pre-reform British system can be hypothesised to be more conducive to efficiency in presenting persons with a home alternative to residential care.

2 Home care in England

The chapter first describes the main features of the British system around service provision, access and assessment. It then describes the evolution of the logic underlying reform proposals and the implementation. Finally, it describes some of the main post-reform features.

1. Main features pre-reform

1.1. Service provision

In contrast with the complexity of the French model, that of England and Wales is structurally simple, particularly prior to the community care reforms of April 1993 and therefore during the period covered by the British part of this study. As a result of a general duty placed upon them by the 1948 National Assistance Act, home help services were provided directly by local authority social services departments, who also provided the other components of related domiciliary social service provision such as day care and meals-on-wheels, often in conjunction with voluntary organisations. The voluntary organisations who undertook this social care provision, however, were normally funded by the local authorities on a block grant basis, which meant that there was little control of the quality or quantity of service provided, except in very general terms. Health-related domiciliary care was provided by the home nursing service of the National Health Service with its own lines of finance and management.

Since both the home help and home nursing services were provided by local or central government monopolies with directly employed staff, the level of supply was primarily determined by the budgetary priorities of the services. Users could not influence supply through an incentive to producers to increase profits. Neither did they have much incentive or opportunity to signal the appropriateness of what they were being provided with by shifting their custom elsewhere. And they did not perceive themselves as having an automatic right to service because of certain clearly-defined qualifying criteria. There was only the possibility of influence through the general democratic process, as well as pressure through organisations such as Age Concern. One had to wait until the introduction of the 1993 community care reforms before the elderly could see themselves as having explicit entitlements. A court case such as that brought by recipients of home care services against their social services department over its reduction of previously agreed levels of service would have been unimaginable at the time of this study in Britain (Laing & Buisson, 1994, p.108).

1.2. Access

In England, one cannot shop around for primary care physicians at public expense until one finds one who will provide a certificate to justify entitlement to a home help. In France, that there is not a standing arrangement for a person to use only one general physician may increase demand for home care as for health services. In other respects, there are fewer supply-side obstacles reducing access to services in England. The financial lines of accountability are simpler and more direct. Prior to the reforms, access to the home help service was by way of the service organiser, who would normally accept referrals from any relevant agency, such as the general practitioner, the district nurse, voluntary organisation, family member or the elderly person themselves. In the same way, access to the home nursing service was through the general practitioner, who was open to referrals from any relevant party. For the services such as meals-on-wheels or day care, however, practice varied widely, with these being accessed via social workers, home help organisers, or even the service organisers themselves, despite the fact that, in many local authorities, the services were provided by voluntary organisations.

This variety in access routes for different services which might be required by the same persons, caused as well as illustrated the lack of effective coordination between the various agencies, each of whom had their own priorities for the resources which they controlled, and could lead to the situation in which the elderly person could be the only person with an overview of all the various inputs, no agency having the responsibility or necessity to coordinate them.

1.3. Assessment: structures and incentives

Home help was financed by local authorities from their own revenue, including the central government general grant. The distribution of the grant between expenditure heads was not determined by the central government, leaving prioritisation to the elected local authorities. The same funds also paid for local authority residential provision. The mechanism called 'joint funding' facilitated to some degree joint work on specific shared goals by the local social services and health authorities. However, the state also provided for persons of low income in private residential care by means of a benefit which did not require social services assessment of dependency and the best means of support. That benefit was not cash-limited. It created an incentive for both health and local authorities to divert demand to this source of funding, in effect using it as a safety valve at a time of fiscal stringency and fixed budgets. The incentive was perverse because the benefit was tied to residential care. It therefore encouraged admission to homes of persons who could have received adequate care in their own homes at substantially lower costs (and with what they would have perceived as a higher quality of life).

Management of the services was weak, both within the social services departments and more broadly. Home care, like social work with elderly people, was seen as a Cinderella service compared with the more prestigious child care social work teams. High proportions of staff lacked training. A report of 1979 for the National Council of Home Help Services put the figure at 40 per cent. At the level of the actual service, organisers were still expected to manage teams of up to 100 home helps, as had been the case since the fifties (Davies, 1968; Gwynne and Fean, 1978). Assessment was crude. A report on the home help service in 1970 (Hunt, 1973) stated: 'practically all the assessments appear to be subjective: only two organisers (out of 54 interviewed) worked to a scale and very few attempted a definition of "needs"'. The same could have been written fifteen years later. This lack of precision over targeting criteria led to increasing dilution of intensity of cover in order to cover a growing demand, and was not monitored against clear outcomes (Davies, 1968; Davies et al., 1990).

The home nursing service, controlled through the general practitioner, had a range of qualified staff. Health visitors allocated about 8 per cent of their time to care of the elderly (White Paper, 1989). They undertook more specialised health assessments on behalf of the GP to whom they were attached. District nurses holding a national state registration would normally undertake skilled interventions, again under the general direction of the GP to whom they were attached. They allocated some 80 per cent of their effort to the elderly. Nursing auxiliaries, who had a lower-level qualification, worked under the supervision of the district nurse to perform tasks associated with personal care, such as washing and bathing. There was some scope for overlap within the health provision, with district nurses often having to undertake the personal care tasks that could have been left to auxiliaries, and nursing services filling gaps left as a result of the under-provision of home help services.

Increasingly during the eighties, authorities attempted to provide for larger numbers of persons at a time of financial stringency by raising more revenue from charges to users. A survey by the Association of Directors of Social Services in 1982 revealed that no less than 42 authorities put up their charges in 1981/2 by over 40 per cent (ADSS, 1982). Evidence about the effect on demand was ambiguous. Some concluded that the level of the charge reduced demand. Others suggested that such an effect was temporary. Yet others inferred that among those who used any home care service, the amount demanded was supply-controlled, unaffected by the charge made on the marginal units, and no less supply-determined among the less rather than more needy (Judge and Matthews, 1980; Evandrou and Winter, 1988; Davies et al., 1990). The charging arrangements presented perverse incentives to all the participants: users, their family caregivers, and agencies.

- Health provision was free, leading to the diversion of demand to home nursing services. Likewise there was a diversion of demand to hospital care. More of the demand was deflected because local authorities were restricting services to cope with tight budgets.
- Among those qualified to receive supplementary benefit (having a low income and savings of below £1,200), there were uncapped social security benefits which fully funded private residential care.

• Those allocating home care services had little incentive to target resources flexibly and efficiently at those who were at high risk of admission to institutions but whose admission was unwanted and unnecessary. This further limited the scope to provide the more flexible responses demanded by those with more unpredictable needs, such as persons suffering cognitive impairment due to Alzheimer's disease. For example, it was difficult to provide carers with flexible and effective relief sitting. (For that reason, such services were developed linked with the hospice movement.) There was little incentive to fill the gap between skilled nursing at home, provided by the health authority, and the narrow range of services provided by the local authority home help services, limited at the most to domestic cleaning and shopping, perhaps supplemented by an intermittent and volunteer-based meals-on-wheels service.

• Attendance allowances paid at one of two levels to those needing help with personal care tasks either for part or all of the day or night had a low ceiling, equivalent to approximately 20 per cent of the cost of residential care. The criteria for targeting were not linked to those for social care. There was no automatic cross-referral of cases of a kind which would allow the social services to provide brokerage to recipients of attendance allowances. Although intended for the procurement of help, there was no mechanism to check that the benefit was even partly used for this service. It came to be seen as a supplement to income rather than as a recompense for the costs associated with disability, and its relevance to funding home care was therefore tenuous.

2. The evolution of the policy

We can usefully distinguish several periods in the recent British history of community care.

2.1. Confluence of policy-shaping influences, 1974-86

The reforms of the nineties were the product of the conjunction of events and ideas of the decade starting in the late seventies. The most powerful forces were those which influenced all public policy, not the critiques of community and long-term care itself, although it was the critique which provided the specific goals and instruments. The critique channelled the broader forces as much as the broader forces adapted the solutions suggested by the critiques.[1]

One such influence was the Oil Crisis and the collapse of growth-focused economic policy, resulting in devaluation, strait-jacketed economic policy, the search for cuts in public expenditure, and the break-up of the basis for cooperation between employers, unions and the government. This was one part of the context in which Rose (1975) and others discussed 'government overload': the increasing ambition of policy aims and the increasing gap between performance and expectations. The performance of the traditional agencies of the local welfare state were challenged from different quarters with criticisms heard first during the sixties. They had much in common, including unresponsiveness to user needs and wishes. By the late seventies, there were academic critiques of inflexibility and targeting in a wide range of policy areas, including community care (Davies, 1981; Goldberg and Connelly, 1982). In health and personal social services policy-making, the initial effect of the turmoil of the mid-seventies was to halt progress in implementing old policies without replacing it with a new long-term strategy.

The failure of corporatism was accompanied by a stream of argument from the 'new right' in policy analysis, 'think tanks' echoing for broad

1 Taking one of the oldest symbols of the welfare state — the school meals service — a case study showed how social change had created variations in need between individuals and so the populations of small areas, and, similarly, variations in the factors causing uptake; how the relative costs of mitigating the nutritional consequences of child poverty differed between small geographical areas; and how the needs were being met with an inappropriately uniform response by authorities. In consequence, the benefits of the large subsidy were not received by proportions for whom they would be of most benefit, and the public money was not spent in the most cost-effective way. In *Universality, Selectivity and Effectiveness in Social Care* (Davies, 1978), it was argued that a solution would be for local managers to be set the task of mitigating the nutritional consequences of child poverty, to be allocated budgets to do so, being held accountable by the examination of outcomes (Davies, 1978). That was an almost identical model to the Kent Community Care Project whose initial design was stated in Davies (1974), save that the allusion to contracting supply was more explicit, and the budget was to be held by field workers.

public consumption the theoretical arguments of American public choice economists and others. The inflexibility and inefficiencies of government were ascribed to the nature of public bureaucracy. Competitive markets were promoted as an alternative, leading to the 'privatisation' of public utilities and enterprises, the creation of autonomous agencies to perform functions hitherto undertaken by government, the reform of the NHS around the purchaser/provider split, and the 'local management of schools'. Accountability through the ballot box in a public bureaucracy was contrasted by Michael Heseltine with accountability to consumers in a market, and the latter was promoted as a better alternative than the former as a principle for reform. Nicholas Ridley, a predecessor to Heseltine as Secretary of State for the Environment (a portfolio which includes responsibility for local government affairs), defined a concept of an 'enabling authority'; not primarily a provider, certainly not the near-monopolist provider, but regulator, sponsor and coordinator, contracting with independent providers for the supply of services for those for whom it has a financial responsibility. The suppliers would operate in a competitive market (Ridley, 1988). Though not clearly articulated in the speech itself, such ideas were circulating among policy-makers and others some years earlier, at the time of the Buxton speech by the Secretary of State for Health and Social Services to directors of social services in 1984 (Fowler, 1984).

However, not all the arguments that the authorities should play more ambitious enabling roles came from the 'new right'. In practice, the arrangements for the social security financing of residential care most stimulated the growth of for-profit provision, not provision by not-for-profit trusts, or traditional or new forms of voluntary organisation. Some authorities considered the flexible purchasing of services to be desirable in some circumstances. The circumstances included the operation of local trade and industry policies, including strict rules of competition to ensure playing fields designed to avoid distortions, and local attempts to develop a wider range of forms of ownership and auspices. Some of the literature sought the clear separation of provision from commissioning and purchasing at the individual and area level for only some services, arguing that, for many users, the benefits from arm's length commissioning of some home care services would be more than offset by the costs of adequate coordination and quality assurance. For some, the emphasis was more on making entry easier for potential providers in order to increase the variety of provision than on eliminating 'producers surpluses' due to inefficiency in the provision of a few relatively homogeneous services. Examples were quoted of such developments in other countries, and the nature of the trade and industry policies which stimulated and moulded them. Such argument saw such arrangements as complementary to, not in opposition to, the best of the development during the Seebohm years and later, particularly if lessons from other countries were properly learned (Davies, 1986; Davies and Challis, 1986; Davies, 1990; Davies et al., 1990).

The Thatcher administration from 1979 believed in the contribution which the styles and techniques of private sector management could introduce to the public sector, and encouraged their application with vigour (Davies, 1988; Pollitt, 1990).

One response to the Financial Management Initiative was the replacement of the Audit Office by the Audit Commission for Local Government, whose focus was broad cost-effectiveness (White Paper, 1983). The Commission did much to introduce the new managerialist ideas to a local government system conditioned by the agenda of the early seventies. The Audit Commission produced powerful critiques of efficiency and effectiveness of community care policy (Audit Commission, 1985, 1986). The Department of Health response was the replacement of the Social Work Service (focused on professional effectiveness, particularly in child welfare) by a Social Services Inspectorate with a duty to promote efficiency as well as effectiveness. By the mid-eighties, some of its inspections were clearly showing the influence of the new academic arguments about failures to match resources to needs in community care, and its effects on the targeting of resources and their impacts on outcomes (Social Services Inspectorate, 1987). Both the Audit Commission and the Social Services Inspectorate were powerful because their writings were so widely studied by managers and policy-makers at the central and local levels. Being inspectorates, both worked to programmes which followed up the impact of their earlier findings about individual agencies.

The term 'new managerialism' was by coincidence used by different scholars to describe two sets of related phenomena. One was the adoption in government generally of some of the values, assumptions and techniques used in private sector management: clear statements of mission; statements of objectives for managers at all levels in concrete terms against short-term time scales fixing their responsibility for the success of the 'cost centres' and 'profit centres'; and the monitoring of performance in addressing objectives using information systems collecting process and outcome information as well as inputs to produce 'the incentivizing of line managers' (Pollitt, 1990, p.56). One could also include concepts of 'total quality management'; more extensive management training; the delegation of authority and responsibility with cash-limited budgets for achieving the goals within a more effective system of accountability so as to encourage resourcefulness and responsiveness — 'a strategy of purposeful opportunism'; and adaptiveness about means with constancy about ends (Klein and O'Higgins, 1985). In that sense, new managerialism was a powerful influence in all government agencies.

The second sense alluded mainly to post-reorganisation local authorities. It was an allusion to local government as a 'political institution constituted for local choice' (Stewart, 1986). To Stewart, the 'new managerialism' was a response to the break-up of the consensus and the spread of party conflict in local government in the years following the reorganisation of 1974. Some progressive authorities had provided some antecedents from the mid-sixties (Friend and Jessup, 1969). Whereas 'learning, choice, flexibility, responsiveness and political control' were all important in the dictionary of Stewart's 'new managerialism' in this second sense, they were not important concepts in the lexicon of new managerialism in its first sense. Reflecting the second 'political' meaning, local authorities were defined as 'public sector organisations, not market organisations', making their decisions 'subject to political control, rather than market discipline' (Stewart, 1986, p.4). This too looked a more doubtful prescription for those areas of activity in which authorities were only some of the providers, and had lost market dominance. Again, the description looked doubtful in their roles as regulators of quality and the commissioners and promoters of supply.

2.2. Model logic and implementation, 1986-1995

This was the second period. It was one when the model was designed and elaborated at the level of principle. The Audit Commission published a pungent critique of community care in 1986. It found an excessive reliance on residential modes of care, a slow creation of community-based services, and an uneven pattern of local provision. It considered that a community-based service could be provided with current levels of expenditure. But it would require rationalisation of funding policy from the centre, a more rational organisational structure with 'local responsibility, authority and accountability for delivering a balanced community-based care services ... more clearly defined', with 'greater managerial authority delegated to the local level'. It concluded that changes were required in the 'organisational framework for community care'. 'In order to establish how best to achieve this end, a high level review of the current situation should be set in train' (Audit Commission, 1986, p.4).

The government response was to invite a report from Sir Roy Griffiths, managing director of J. Sainsbury, the chain of grocery supermarkets; the model legislated in most essential respects was the set of arrangements proposed by the Griffiths report (1988).

The Griffiths model

The model was based on six elements. The distributions of functions implied are summarised in Box 1.

Box 1. The Griffiths model

- The consolidation of authority, responsibility and accountability for policy and practice decisions and for financing their consequences
- A clearer focus on community care policy-making and management by the DH
- Concentration of responsibility for (i) 'trade and industry' policy functions and (ii) the performance of the 'core tasks of case management' and its management on local lead agencies.
- Focusing the LASSD on these responsibilities, and away from direct provision.
- Focusing public subsidies on the poor.
- Concentrating responsibility for performing the core tasks of case management and the management of their performance.

• *The consolidation of authority, responsibility and accountability for policy and practice decisions and for financing their consequences.* This was the central principle. In the words of the report: 'a budgetary approach) centrally and locally, which aligns responsibility for achieving objectives with control over the resources needed to achieve them so that therc is a built-in incentive and the facility to make the best use of the resources available'.[2] (Griffiths, 1988, para. 5.6). 'The absence of such processes at the national level is inconsistent with any claim that there are serious national objectives to be achieved' (para. 5.7).

This 'fundamental' element of the logic of the report required, it argued, a suitable financial system. The distorting effects of the then system were among the most publicised of the problems of community care. These pernicious effects of the arrangements had been described with eloquence and power in many well-researched analyses. In particular, there was the failure of devices to overcome the separation of the funding of long-term social as distinct from nursing and medical care in hospitals (particularly in psychiatric hospitals); and the social security benefit for residence in for-profit rest homes, a subsidy which had increased from £10 million in 1980 to £1.5 billion by 1993.[3] But not all of the effects have been traced in the literature: for instance, the consequences for the creation and then destruction of promising new modes of care.[4] Mechanisms for financing care (and fiscal mechanisms generally) can helpfully be used to provide incentives to equity and

2 'Such a system will facilitate effective planning and responsiveness to change. It is self-evident that resources must be consistent with the agreed responsibilities and objectives to be achieved within a given timescale.' 'A similar approach is needed both at local and national levels to ensure that the entire resources allocated are properly identified and accounted for' (para. 5.6).

3 A junior minister suggested in parliamentary debate that the use of the social security benefit to create a for-profit sector during the eighties was deliberate, however accidental was its genesis.

4 An example was adult fostering/boarding out. Its value has been shown in the Oregon evaluation (Kane, 1988). It is a case which illustrates two impor- tant features of the problem: first, how the old DHSS guidelines changed benefit structures and regulations to kill off undesired supplier responses which had been stimulated by incentives caused by changes in social security arrangements; and second, how the responses of suppliers were (and are) accelerating, this in turn inviting a faster response from the DHSS.

efficiency. But to achieve this, they must be simple, stable and enduring. That is a lesson still to be fully learnt by the British local authorities (Davies, 1989).

• A diagram in the White Paper was to show the budget of the local authority social services department (LASSD) being allocated from its headquarters to field case management teams, only at that level it being allocated to providers in the form of purchases of services (White Paper, 1989, Chart 7).

• *A clearer focus on community care policy-making and management by the Department of Health.* The focus of the Audit Commission report was local: the fragmentation of responsibility and accountability and the distortions in incentives, not the weaknesses in the policy machine at the Department of Health. Griffiths focused on the centre, echoing a theme of questioning by new Tory MPs of Department of Health spokesmen to the House of Commons Social Services Committee in 1990, a theme subsequently not pursued by the Committee as they became acclimatised to the cultures of the community care world (Davies and Challis, 1986, pp.516-19). It was necessary to have articulated policy around 'the budgetary approach, centrally and locally', backed by the determination to implement it successfully in order to mobilise the energy, stimulate the imagination, and raise the morale of officials; and provide the criteria needed to commission and organise work in a way that it would have the greatest benefit to the outside world. The implications of the Griffiths discussion was that the DHSS should be more directive and managerial, removing the last vestiges of the 'laissez-faire' assumptions of the old Ministry of Health (Griffiths, 1988).

Griffiths recommended that there should be a Minister of State for Community Care: an Alexandrine prince who would cut the Gordian knots of the existing system.

Central government should have a greater 'direct stake ... in the delivery of its policies at the local level' (para. 5.12).[5] He therefore

5 It required that stake 'not just because of the intrinsic national importance of those policies, but also because of the considerable interrelationships between what is done by local authorities, and what may or may not need to be done by others more directly accountable to central government, and in particular by health authorities' (para. 5.12). The specific grants would be necessary to recognise the interdependence of local and central government programmes; to provide a degree of central government influence and

recommended specific grants for the financing of community care, not the general grant for all local authority purposes. That was not put into effect. However, the large transitional grant from 1993 has been specific.

• *Concentration of responsibility for (i) 'trade and industry' policy functions and (ii) the performance of the 'core tasks of case management' and its management on local lead agencies.* Griffiths did not use the term 'trade and industry policy', but it is more resonant than some of the alternative concepts. Using it helps to extend the discourse about the range of interventions, to reflect the need to be proactive and not merely reactive, and to provide the unifying purpose for them: the prevention or correction of failures of an unmanaged market (Davies, 1986, 1990). It is a much wider concept than preventing a shortfall from minimum standards for those users least able to assert themselves and demand adequate standards. There is a case for assessing the potential of some trade and industry policy for any area relying on markets for allocation in producing less than equitable outcomes or producing them inefficiently. The study of trade and industry policies in existing mixed economies, for instance in Australia or such states as New York, illustrates that the scope of trade and industry policies in current British policy is narrow. In the USA also, it was concluded that payment for care in facilities should be linked to dependency level. In the UK, practice varies between local authorities; some invite tenders. This has not led to the escalation of fees as occurred in, for instance, New York during the seventies (Moreland Commission, 1975). The contrast is that, in the USA, Medicaid has had to compete in a 'seller's market' with great pressure of demand on places. In the UK, there has been a 'buyer's market', with empty beds in many facilities. So the British local authority buyer has been able to obtain low prices. Whether or not it is a 'buyer's' or 'seller's' market for care is crucial to the consequences of choosing one rather than another method of purchasing.

• *Focusing the LASSD on these responsibilities, and away from direct provision.* The Griffiths report also talked about the enabling authority. 'The primary function of the public services is to design and arrange the provision of care and support in line with people's needs. That care

---

control; to create a more stable basis for planning and delivery of services; and to ensure transferred funds reach their intended destination' (para. 5.14).

and support can be provided from a variety of sources. There is value in a multiplicity of provision, ... because of the widening of choice, creativity, innovation and competition it should stimulate. It is vital that social services authorities should see themselves as the arrangers and purchasers of care services — not as monopolistic providers.'

• *Focusing public subsidies on the poor.* 'It seems right that those able to pay the full economic cost of community care services should be expected to do so'.

• *Concentrating responsibility for performing the core tasks of case management and the management of their performance.* Griffiths calls this 'a keystone' of his proposals. He proposed that a case manager should be assigned wherever 'a significant level of resources' was expected (para. 6.6), or where the case was complex. The concentration of responsibility is associated with the intention to 'align responsibility for achieving objectives with control over the resources needed to achieve them, so that there is a built-in incentive and the facility to make the best use of the resources available' (para. 5.6). It is a small minority of case manage- ment programmes in the USA and elsewhere which do this in a way which gives the case manager the preconditions for behaving flexibly, resourcefully and responsively to the needs and wishes of clients and informal carers (Davies, 1992). However, Griffiths had seen the British programmes which did this, and took some trouble to learn about the argument and experience.

The White Paper version

The White Paper in most essential respects followed the Griffiths model. It weakened the link between budgeting at the centre and the local authorities by not ensuring that all the long-term care money released in the health services was transferred to local authorities for community care. It was shown that the greater part of the cost of the Bérégovoy proposals for the French *prestation — autonomie — dépendance* would have been to remove inequalities between departments: the budget for *'péréquation'* (Chombeau, 1992). Articulation of the budget at central and local levels might have put pressure on the Treasury to face similar tax costs in the UK.

The White Paper fitted the approach to community care into a theme of the administration running through all areas of social policy: 'choice and independence', by 'enabling people to live as normal a life as possible in their own homes or in a homely environment in the local community, providing the right amount of care and support to help people achieve maximum possible independence ..., and giving people a greater individual say in how they live their lives and the services they need to help them to do so.'

The objectives of policy were therefore (i) to develop domiciliary day and respite services to enable people to live in their own homes wherever feasible and sensible; (ii) to ensure that service providers make practical support for carers a high priority; (iii) to make proper assessment of need and good case management the cornerstone of high-quality care; (iv) to promote the development of a flourishing independent sector alongside good-quality public services, making maximum possible use of private and voluntary providers; (v) to clarify the responsibilities of agencies and so make it easier to hold them to account for their performance; and (vi) to secure better value for taxpayers' money by introducing a new funding structure for social care, removing the incentive to use residential and nursing home care rather than care in the home. The changes were:

- SSDs became responsible, in collaboration with workers from other agencies, for assessing individual need, designing care arrangements, and securing their delivery within available resources: that is, perform care management tasks within a budget. A responsibility was placed on the health authorities to make the necessary contributions to multidisciplinary procedures.
- SSDs produced and published plans consistent with health authority plans, which were to be inspected by the Department of Health, and the health authorities were expected to prepare community care plans.
- SSDs were exhorted, and given powerful financial incentives, to make the maximum use of the independent sector, securing services under contracting and making other arrangements for financial support of provision, and in other ways 'promoting the mixed economy of care' (para. 3.4.6). To make the competition between suppliers from different sectors fairer, it advocated an organisational separation of the performance of some of the tasks: care management and its management, the supply of services, the sponsorship and development of supply and service providers, and the quality assurance of services.
- SSDs took on the responsibility for financing community care.

• SSDs were required to establish inspection and registration units at arm's length from the management of their own services to check standards in both their own homes and independently-owned homes. They were to establish user complaints and inspection procedures and to publicise them.

• A new specific grant was introduced to aid the development of social care for seriously mentally ill people.

The White Paper stated the intention to nominate a care manager where an individual's needs were complex or significant levels of resources were involved (para. 3.3.2), and saw advantage in linking care management with delegated responsibility for budgetary management (para. 3.3.5). LASSDs were expected to show in their care plans how they proposed to apply case management techniques.

Policy guidance

The Department of Health made a distinction between 'what is expected of ... authorities' to conform to policy, and how the policy should be implemented. Policy guidance (Department of Health, 1990) was the 'what' document: the statement of the policy content particularly with respect to structure and process: 'the framework within which the delivery of community care should be planned, developed, commissioned and implemented locally' (para. 1.4).

In effect, it focused on what the Department of Health considered to be all the key areas and tasks for the implementation (para. 1.4). Among other areas, it covered community care plans; care management and assessment of individuals' needs; commissioning and purchasing from independent providers; independent inspection units for quality assessment; user complaints procedures; and the mental illness care programme approach and specific grant.

The policy logic in its context

The accounts in this chapter have shown how the policy proposals blended the logics of the elements described earlier. It exploited the structural consolidation of political responsibility, authority and accountability at national and local levels and in important respects enhanced it. It made the vaguer ambitions of the sixties into concrete goals. It put into effect the lessons of the first type of new managerialist argument. It created a version of the enabling authority concept, and pressed the mixing of the supply economy of care with great determination and powerful new rewards and sanctions. It created the surrogate consumer — the user-/carer-responsive care manager — to be the personal broker for cases for which that would yield the greatest benefits. It pressed for services to carers, and pressed for changes to empower users and carers. It advocated that authorities move at the speed they could muster, giving them control over the public funds to balance the interests of their caseload as a group against that of individuals within the limits of their budgets, so providing the care managers with an incentive continually to improve cost-effectiveness in the use of public funds. It was more explicit in its abandonment of some of the vague universalism of the sixties. It created the first essentials of a 'trade and industry' policy to develop and avoid disbenefits in the new market structures.

Implementation

The new policy was implemented in stages from 1991. The changes have been vast. The research evaluations have so far produced evidence about process rather than about outcomes for users, the family caregivers, and the equity and efficiency in the use of resources.

3. Post-reform features

• *The consolidation of responsibility between agencies has clarified issues.* However, the interdependence of the demand for health and social care is increasing not only because the services are increasingly targeted at the more dependent, but also because of changes in medical technology itself. Therefore, far more of the demands for community social care in the mid-nineties are for short-term care during 'post-acute' periods, and the degree to which the goals of each agency are achieved is much more dependent on the resources provided by other agencies, particularly health and housing. This trend is causing the redefinition of the roles of services which may come to be reflected in a redefinition of the roles of agencies. There has been a tendency for the perception of issues to be limited to their narrow manifestations, not sufficiently working through the contradictions between underlying changes in technologies, structures and assumptions. The need to respond has distracted from some of the longer-term investments in the components of the policy logic. For example, incontinence has become more treatable and/or manageable, but care managers have little training, and practice protocols have not been developed for them or providers for its handling to best effect in the local contexts. The same is so for depression (Banerjee, 1996). Few care managers and providers in providing agencies are trained to identify the iatrogenic consequences of drug regimens made inappropriate by quick changes in health circumstances. They do not work *with* physicians and others to monitor the signs and symptoms of changes in the diseases — or in the consequences of the diseases — for which a diagnosis has already been made for their cases; and they are not trained to look more generally for the signs and symptoms of common diseases of old age. It is not just that interdisciplinary working in multidisciplinary multi-agency teams have not developed quickly for the users for whom the costs would be most worthwhile: for instance, the medically unstable with some conditions and circumstances. It is that collaboration — the exchange of information and cooperation — is insufficiently widespread and reliable.

• *The dominance of independent providers in the economy of shelter-with-care has been consolidated.* The position of the independent providers has been consolidated. Independent residential and nursing home care provision accounted for 79 per cent and independent daycare provision for 19 per cent of their respective SSD-brokered markets in 1996 (Department of Health, 1997a,b). Because of continuous central government pressure and incentives, the market share of independent providers in home care had grown by September 1996 to 36 per cent (Department of Health, 1997b). The growth in home care has been more limited in some other countries which are seeking to mix the supply economy of care: for example, Sweden. Successive investigations of the structure of the economy of care suggest that recent changes in policies and assumptive worlds among the senior managers have been greater than are reflected in the actual distribution of market share during the nineties (Kendall and Knapp, 1995; Wistow et al., 1994, 1996).

• *The introduction of care management has resulted in a wide variety of models, but only a small proportion of the population live in areas with models which have all the features promoted in the guidelines provided by the Department of Health.* The emphasis of the earlier care management tasks and process have played their part in complementing the increased variety of provision of home and community services, and the range of expenditure on each case has much increased. The earliest results of the study commissioned to evaluate the impact of the changes on who benefits in what way and at what costs to whom, illustrate the key importance of the perceptions of the case managers (Davies et al., 1995; Davies and Fernández, 1997). However, the failure to apply and build on enough of the features from the British experiments was a serious mistake. In consequence:

- Care management effort and resources are being seriously wasted in most authorities by being spread too thinly. There is a big gap between the perceptions and discourse of most SSD managers designing care management arrangements and the academic writing summarising evidence-based argument from around the world about what care management arrangements would match user circumstances, policy priorities, and local system circumstances.
- The interpretation of the policy of giving greater priority in resource allocation to those in greater need has been too narrowly interpreted. There is excessive focus on functional dependence. Those responsibilities seem not to have absorbed the results from the care management experiment that some of the highest ratios of gain to cost from care management and social care packages tend to be made from the careful targeting of inexpensive packages for selected users of lower disability. The targeting of case management in the first generation of American social and health maintenance organisations has been criticised for being unrelated to medical decision-making and planning for health-related as well as social services, and for failing to target at those who had high-risk conditions, evidence of impending disability or high risk of hospitalisation established by annual medical-social assessments (Kane et al., 1997). The post-reform application has so far biased the receipt of any service at all against these circumstances.
- The case management arrangements put in place by British social services departments seem (from the evidence as yet available) to have caused a serious waste of resources, and so, given fixed service supply, the exclusion of needy cases. There are at least four reasons.

  (i) In most authorities the budgets which cover the whole costs of the package of closely complementary and substitute services have not been delegated to the team, and neither are there budget limits which total team costs for all cases must not exceed. That removes from care managers the incentive to consider the opportunity cost of marginal spending in relation to the benefit on each case. Indeed, many care managers do not have clear information on costs and prices.

(ii) Authorities frequently do not have valid and full information on costs appropriately computed — including, for instance, an appropriate apportionment for overheads and capital allowances and covering the whole range of resource flows. The figures in their accounts systematically understate the unit costs of services.

(iii) The cost figures produced are for average not marginal costs, and average prices not the price of an additional unit. The local supply curves for most services, community-based as well as residential, are elastic; that is, a unit additional to the quantity consumed has a higher-than-average price (Davies et al., 1990; Audit Commission, 1996). It is the price of the additional (marginal) unit which is more likely to approximate to the opportunity cost of that unit of service. The difference is particularly critical for making the best use of resources.

(iv) The systematic management review of databases describing team performance in terms of (a) targeting care management; (b) unit costs of cases through time; and (c) outcomes packages is an important prerequisite for equity and efficiency. Such systems were developed for the Kent Community Care Project and further developed when the model was implemented in each area of Kent during the subsequent seven years. *Matching Resources to Needs* (Davies and Challis, 1986) discussed the requirement in the context of professional and management review procedures in the USA. Initially, the database was designed for the analysis of resources, needs and outcomes. This approach partly reflected how the Americans had tackled the design of collections, and partly reflected the focus of the PSSRU's production of welfare approach. Later, the repeated assessment of needs-related circumstances was replaced by a review more orientated to ends and means in social work practice. This more practice- and process-focused approach was modelled on the instrumentation work of E.M. Goldberg (Goldberg and Warburton, 1979). That contributed little to external managerial and professional review, and detracted from the capacity to analyse changes in needs-related circumstances through time. The practice — and process-focused component is not commonly part of current British systems. But neither, unfortunately, is the systematic external managerial review of team targeting, and changes in individual need, unit costs, and outcomes. One reason may be that it was not stressed in the Department of Health guidance (1990).

• *There has been a substantial shift in public subsidy towards the poorer and more dependent, reflecting changes in charging policies as well as in professionally-dominated allocation of services. The balance between demands and resources has been geographically uneven and temporally volatile.* At first, the increase in public expenditure outran the growth of demand created by, in effect, removing the age-old 'workhouse test' which limited demand in all countries in which intensive care could only be obtained in residential institutions for long-term care at the price of a loss of autonomy and an admission of defeat.[6] That, and the failure of authorities to balance the expansion and increased user-responsiveness of care with controls on targeting, continued in some authorities but, in others, the subsequent allocations of the special grant from the central government to support the implementation of the reform were less favourable, while demand responded to the more attractive services, causing disruption. The result has been to disrupt the progress in some of the most ambitious authorities most committed to some of the central ideas of the new policy.

6 The 'workhouse test' was imposed following the Local Government Reform Act of 1832. The Act was a response to the escalation in the costs of poor relief during the previous fifty years, due to the use of poor relief to subsidise low wages. The logic of the Act was to force persons seeking poor relief to enter 'the workhouse', a residential institution in which the level of living and the nature of the regime were intended to be sufficiently unattractive to deter all but the most desperate.

3 Home care in France

Variety and diversity between areas are as much a feature of French care provision as of French cuisine. In 1992 'one département had 60 different home help services, and 180 communes, each with its own allocation priorities' (comment made at a study day organised by Fondation de France, 1992). In Dunquerque, one home help service alone had 42 sources of finance in 1990. Perhaps this fragmentation and complexity is one reason why the literatures describing the French system so often combine description of the legal and financial base of services with some statistics and a critique of its overall functioning, without detailed analysis of structure, content and process at the field levels. The description given in next section will do no more than sketch the range of services and their formal purpose. Later sections will mention themes of the critique.

1. Principal services

The modern system was developed after the publication of the Laroque report in 1962 (Inspection générale des affaires sociales, 1962). Prior to that, families were responsible under the principle of *obligation alimentaire*, those without a family being helped by public assistance, non-profit organisations employing home helps, or residential facilities, principally public assistance institutions. The Laroque report conceived the policy goal for elderly persons to be to support them as autonomous, actively participating persons of the third age, integrated into the community and supported to live independently in their own homes wherever possible. To achieve the goal, it would be necessary to develop a range of services and other interventions to tackle housing problems, stimulate social activity, and provide help with household chores and nursing needs. However, the main development occurred only from the early seventies.

1.1. Home help

The home help service was provided for by legislation in 1962. The collective agreement coming into force in 1983 confirmed its purpose to be to enable persons to remain in their own homes. It was both to be an adjunct of home nursing and to be available without medical justification to those at risk of admission to an institution for long-term care. Initially financed by the *assurance maladie* (sickness benefit), the provision of home help was linked with old age insurance when that was separated in 1967.

Occurring from that time, the development was caught up in the policy of decentralisation, with the *départements* (higher tier local authorities) allocating the services. Against a background of pressure on budgets, authorities tended to spend so as to affect the largest number of persons (Guillemard, 1986). The same tendency occurred in the home help service, leading to the problem of *sapoudrage* (a sprinkling), as it was called by the Schopflin report (1991).

Financing

For persons aged 65 and over, of low income, and who live alone or with a person unable to undertake the activities, there is a statutory financial benefit, *aide sociale.* The service is provided by the municipalities. A recipient can obtain up to 30 hours per month. *Assurances vieillesse* and the *régimes spéciaux* whose primary task is to finance pensions also finance home help, although each scheme determines the eligibility criteria and other benefit rules. (We have mentioned the variation in policies earlier in this section.) The cover is the same for those financed either by public assistance or covered by the general scheme for salaried and industrial workers, *Caisse national d'assurance vieillesse* (CNAV).

Supply

There are two main types of service provision. The first, and simplest to identify from an English standpoint, is where the home helps are employed by the commune and operate as local authority employees. However, this is not the usual model in France. Rather, the service is organised by *associations* established as not-for-profit organisations according to the laws of 1 July 1901 and 16 August 1901, which define the status and method of financial and fiscal accountability of voluntary organisations.

Within this general framework, the *association* typically acts as organiser, assessor and employer, within terms defined by the financing agencies by means of a *Convention*. However, newer types of *association*, called *mandataire*, are developing in France which act either partly as employers of home helps, and partly as brokers or, in the case of some *associations*, solely as brokers. By brokers in this context is meant an organisation which does not employ home helps but, to some greater or lesser extent, helps the elderly person themselves to employ the home help directly. This reflects moves by central government to give fiscal incentives to individuals to employ private help.

Another type of *association* that can be found is one which provides both home help and nursing care (*Associations de soins et service à domicile*, ASSAD). In France, the traditional model of providing home nursing is for the patient to approach a self-employed nurse (*infirmière libérale*), after having obtained a medical certificate from their doctor. The fees of the nurse are then claimed back from the health insurance scheme at the local *Caisse primaire d'assurance maladie* (CPAM). With these new type of home care *associations*, block funding, on a per capita basis, is negotiated from the CRAM (*Caisse régionale d'assurance maladie*) and then allocated by the *association*, according to rules laid down by the convention with the CRAM, to meet home nursing but not home help needs.

Within the period of the study, funds were made available by the main pension scheme, *Caisse nationale d'assurance vieillesse*, CNAV, to pay for non-nursing care out of normal hours. This care, known as *garde à domicile*, includes auxiliary nursing care such as bathing or more typical home help tasks such as preparing meals, and is aimed at bridging the gap between classic nursing and home help tasks, and covering home care needs at night or weekends when normal services are at best only limited. However, such was the demand that, in one of the sites in this study, services had to be withdrawn halfway through the year because the available budget had been spent, and it took much ingenuity by the workers to cover this sudden gap in provision.

1.2. Other services

There was growth in the provision of clubs and restaurants during the seventies. During the eighties, there was an increased emphasis on alternatives to hospitalisation, reflected in the circular issued by the Ministry of Social Affairs and National Solidarity (1986). The intention was to shift resources to socio-medical institutions and day and nursing care. From 1986, a new theme emerged: the creation of employment of persons with few qualifications at danger of social marginalisation. Measures were introduced bypassing the traditional services and facilitating the creation of *associations intermédiaire* whose purpose was to provide cleaners to elderly persons, exempting those aged 70 and over from paying social contributions.

Regulations for the home nursing services were issued in a circular of October 1981, which made the services a priority, defined its objectives, and specified its operating conditions. The objective is to prevent, postpone or shorten stays in hospital and other institutions for long-term care. The service was to provide personal care as well as technical nursing, and was to give more continuous service than the *infirmières libérales*. The service is run by either public or private bodies from a variety of locations. The financing is by the *assurances maladie*, and is provided under a level of service contract with the agency. There are large variations in provision between areas. The service is dominated by tasks associated with the performance of activities of daily living. The service is reported to be well targeted.

1.3. Access

Access to service is by a variety of routes and this posed a problem for the study as it is not easy to ensure that one is collecting data on home care recipients from a single focal point.

One of the closest to the pre-reform English model is by an applicant for publicly funded domiciliary care making contact with the local social services office, the *Centre communal d'action sociale* (CCAS). This is likely either to handle the application itself, or to refer on to the local *association*, or deal with financial eligibility only and then refer on to a local *association* for service assessment and/or provision; which course is followed depends on local practice. From a British perspective, this would seem to resemble a social work role. However, it seems that many CCAS staff see themselves in a more bureaucratic role, dealing mainly with the processing of the relevant application or financial forms. With aims like the more client-oriented approach of a British social services casework model, projects have therefore been undertaken over the past five years, in various localities, to facilitate coordination. They help the elderly person to handle various local agencies to realise an agreed assessment of need on a wider than service-orientated approach. One such project was involved in this study.

Another route for application is to the local office of the applicant's pension fund. This tends to be used mainly where one fund has a concentration of pensioners in a given area such as rural communes, where the *mutualité sociale agricole* (MSA) may well have a call-office for its local social worker in main villages. This would initiate the application, possibly handle the financial assessment, and then refer on to a home help service for needs assessment and/or service provision. For the purposes of this study, however, this would have limited data on applicants to specific employment-based categories of older people, and so was felt to be inappropriate.

In other localities, application can be made direct to the local home help service, who will handle both financial and needs assessment and arrange service delivery. In rural areas, volunteers are often used for some of these tasks, acting as a local point of referral, in monitoring service delivery, assisting in the collection of financial contributions and even, in emergencies out of office hours, organising an immediate response to sudden changes of need. The unified home help and home nursing services (ASSAD) are described in reports such as that of the Schopflin Commission (1991) as being a good model for service delivery. (One of the collaborators in this study is such a service.)

The last main source of information about people applying for publicly-funded home care is the *départemental* social services, who administer the applications for help funded by *aide sociale* for those who lack access to pension fund sources of domiciliary care. The *département* which collaborated in this study had the extra advantage of actively pursuing the funding of domiciliary care by means of a cash allowance, the *Allocation compensatrice pour tierce personne* (ACTP) which the recipients are free to use as they wish to purchase home care, either paying family members or by employing a private help and perhaps benefiting from the government's fiscal incentives to do so.

1.4. Assessment: structures and incentives

At whichever point in the access route the financial assessment is undertaken, it is done on the basis of nationally defined criteria. These criteria are set annually by the funding agencies, either the departmental *aide sociale*, or the various *caisses de retraite*: either those *caisses* which are part of the national social security regimes, or the supplementary schemes (*retraite complémentaire*).

As examples of the tariff of means-tested contributions valid for the period of this study, for those with insufficient monthly income (below 4,539F for a single pensioner,7,886F for a couple), it is possible for *aide sociale* to pay for the home help costs to a maximum of 30 hours per month. Help given by *aide sociale* is recoverable from the estate of recipients, but no contribution is expected from children or other family members under the terms of *obligation alimentaire*.

For those who do not qualify for *aide sociale*, with monthly incomes up to 10,115F/15,221F[1] respectively, the *Caisse nationale d'assurance vieillesse* (CNAV) will help towards home help costs. Other *caisses* follow similar lines, but of course each *caisse* will only pay for those who are their pension recipients.

Service assessment is similarly subject to rules laid down by the funding agencies, and will therefore vary. Some *départements* require a medical certificate, others do not. All limit the number of hours that can be financed; an average is that of the CNAV which is 30 hours per month, or exceptionally up to 90 hours per month maximum. However, this figure could be more or less generous depending on the funding agencies involved, or the living unit of the applicant. (Those in sheltered housing may only qualify for a maximum of 15 or 20 hours per month for example, although the CNAV Circulaire 46/95 of 12 June 1995 seeks to re-align this with other domiciliary settings.) For clients who qualify for *aide sociale* funding, following financial assessment by the

1 As at 01/01/98, Circulaires CNAV nos 15/98 and 16/98 of 18 February 1998.

departmental social services, needs assessment and service allocation is done at local *commune* level, by the *Maire* or CCAS staff. The upper limit varies by *département*, usually within a range of 15 to 30 hours per month. But the financing agency, the *département*, at least in some areas, does not seem to have a systematic way of monitoring the decisions of the communes within that maximum.

All help is limited to non-medical tasks, and need is assessed on ability or otherwise to perform a number of tasks of daily living as follows:

- walk alone;
- manage stairs;
- eat unaided;
- prepare meals;
- lift items such as shopping, coal scuttle, and so on; and
- manage tasks: bed-making, housework, shopping.

There is currently much emphasis on the development of more standardised assessment instrumentation (Colvez et al., 1995). It has been a focus of the experimentation which preceded the preparation of the *projet de loi* (white paper) on the *prestation autonomie*, the proposed benefit which was replaced in favour of *prestation specifique dépendance*. The standard national instrumentation has been criticised for its excessive emphasis on dependency compared with social support (Colvez, 1997; see also ORSMIP, 1993).

Periodic reports criticised the failure to make a reality of the proposals to achieve the support for persons in their own homes required to avoid unnecessary and unwanted admissions to institutions for long-term care, particularly *Vieillir demain* (Commissariat général du plan, 1981). Criticisms mounted during the late eighties, culminating in three reports: the Braun report (Braun and Stourm, 1988), the Boulard report (Assemblé nationale, 1991) and the Schopflin report (1991).

2. Official critique and policy themes

As in the UK, but perhaps later by several years, official reports increasingly drew attention to shortfalls in the performance of the system. From this developing critique one can discern several general themes.

Section 2.1 summarises some of the important criticisms. Section 2.2 states some of the themes.

By the nineties, reform-supporting opinion focused on, *inter alia*, the following criticisms.

• *Aide ménagère* is badly targeted. The average number of hours is low, though rising (Schopflin, 1991, p.55). The service is not targeted primarily at the most dependent. The service is neither sufficiently technical to affect the health status of the elderly person, nor sufficiently flexible in its deployment to permit large inputs and help with the essential acts of daily living even if, in practice, helpers undertake them to some degree. Rules forbid certain tasks. (This is so in the UK, but possibly to a lesser degree.) The attempts of CNAV and the Ministry of Social Affairs to target more at those of higher dependency were thwarted by the regulations. The Schopflin report concluded that *'l'orientation vers le soutien aux plus dépendantes apparait impraticable sans réforme profonde du système'* (Schopflin, 1991, pp.55-57).

• The lack of coordination of the utilisation of the main financing mechanism for the most disabled, *allocation compensatrice*, with that for other recipients of home care. The assessment for *allocation compensatrice* by the COTOREP and financing by the *département* both undermines the responsibility of the local authorities, and also causes delays. The high cost of this benefit fits badly with the attempt of the authorities to reduce spending on *aide sociale*. There are anomalies with respect to *obligation alimentaire* and *récuperation sur succession*, which further complicate incentives. Most financing agencies do not permit the receipt of both *aide ménagère* and *allocation compensatrice*.

• The Schopflin report (1991, p.61) described a *'logique d'émiettement et de cumul'*, and drew from it the need for efficient care management arrangements. It is recognised that the large number of services and other forms of intervention can result in a vast variety of combinations, and with it the fact that *'une même resultat peut être atteint avec des ressources humaines et des coûts très différents dans des contextes très divers'* (Schopflin, 1991, p.60). Also recognised is that there are big differences in the outcomes of resources given complex need-related circumstances, including the nature of the important emotional support[2] and the

2 *'Quels que soient les divers contenus techniques des prestations médico-sociales, leur caractéristique principale est d'avoir un très fort contenu relationnel'*

'production domestique de soins', which is itself influenced by the incentives created by the system of formal intervention. Linked with this is the recognition of the fragmentation and number of services, with resulting gaps. These and the professional motivation of providing professionals result in the extension of provision by the addition of new services, innovation by *sédimentation*, with an emphasis on increasing provision rather than a matching of resources to needs. Workers have the incentive to obtain as much service as they can, since there is no incentive for them to make the most efficient use of resources. There is a tendency to overprescribe rather than produce an effective and efficient overall care plan: *'un projet de vie et de soins'*. The complexity makes simple allocation formulae a doubtful instrument for improving effectiveness and efficiency: *'cette importance réduit à néant l'idée de normer la délivrance des prestations'*. Generally, these characteristics create a sector 'in search of coordination'. More specifically, *'l'existence d'un interlocuteur qualifié pour la personne âgée elle-même et sa famille, qui soit susceptible, le cas échéant, d'organiser la prise en charge et de discuter de ses modalités, est un point essentiel du dispositif'* (Commissariat géneral du plan, 1991, p.62).

• Failure to coordinate at levels other than that of the field makes the system ineffective. Because divisions of labour remain unclarified, there is the duplication of activities, wasteful competition, and gaps; assessment information is inadequate; periods of transition between modes of care are inadequately planned; and there are delays, as in the operation of the cumbersome COTOREP procedures.

• There is a complete separation between home care and care in residential facilities, so the resources of facilities are not easily redeployed externally. Residential institutions are less used to provide respite care by means of day centres and short stays than in other countries. Medium-stay wards do not provide a follow-up service for supporting persons at home, and so tend to become ante-chambers for long-stay wards.

• Training is insufficient for complex cases in home care. Professionals each apply their own perspective. They have little training in team work and little understanding of the contribution of others. General physicians working in a fee-for-service system have few incentives to

---

(Schopflin, 1991, p.63).

care for complex elderly cases: one reason for the tendency to 'medicalise' need. Administrators tend to define needs around administrative categories (Henrard et al., 1990).

2.1. Policy themes

The general policy objective of maintaining people in their own homes for as long as possible has been stated in official reports for over thirty years; from the Laroque Commission of 1962, periodically during the seventies and eighties to the present day.[3] However, the emphasis of development at the local level is on such goals as making services more flexible, improving coordination (sometimes by providing a single point of access), improving personal care services linked to home nursing, better integrating home and residential provisions at the level of the recipient, and achieving greater coherence in budgetary policies and speedier responses, particularly by the COTOREP over decisions on ACTP payments (Schopflin, 1991).

There are incentives to close the gap between a national rhetoric of developing home care in order to reduce the dependence on care in institutions, and providing more general developmental foci at the local level.

---

3 The commitment was clearly central to the position of candidates' policies for long-term care during the election campaign of 1995. President Chirac (1995, pp.10-11) made a response about the necessity of a *prestation-dépendance,* linking it to the overall goal of giving citizen choice of, and in, home care:

Pour les moins autonomes de nos aînés, il faudra créer sans attendre .... une allocation spécifique, dite de dépendance, qui leur permette de choisir, librement et dans la dignité, l'hébergement qu'ils souhaitent. L'insuffisance des moyens actuels, en particulier pour le maintien à domicile, l'inégalité des conditions de prise en charge, selon les départements, sont incompatibles avec les exigences de la solidarité et de l'égalité des droits.

Edouard Balladur's response was

Je m'engage a créer ... une allocation de libre choix pour le maintien à domicile des personnes âgées. Elle leur permettra de faire face aux charges liées a la dépendance, et donc de continuer à vivre chez elles le plus longtemps possible si elles le souhaitent (Balladur, 1995, p.11).

One focus is the influence of user expectations and the incentives facing agencies cooperating in developing *plans gérontologique*. The local collaborators are agencies which compete for users' custom. The application of the principle of *obligation alimentaire* provides powerful incentives to families to seek to maintain persons at home. Families are perceived to have an obligation to help their elderly members remain at home. They are penalised if the relative goes into institutional care. Payments made under *aide sociale* to finance domiciliary care are only subject to *récuperation sur succession*, a claim on the recipient's estate after death. However, if the person enters residential care, a wide range of family members is liable to pay for that care if the person lacks her own means so to do. Thus the system is not financially neutral as between home and residential care. Whether this incentive has much effect will be illuminated by the evidence analysed later in this study.

Assessment

The tools used to rate whether qualifying criteria for services are met must be compatible with the goal of using home care services as a means to divert demand from residential care, if that is the principal aim.[4] Tools vary in the degree to which the condition is met. Systems in which long-term care services developed from health services reflect their history in the emphasis of their assessment instrumentation as much as in who tends to perform what task.[5] Instrumentation tends to put more emphasis on information for (and about) medical and nursing treatment. Functional impairment is covered, though not generally made

---

4 Traditions die hard. In the United States, for a decade, the emphasis of proposals to Congress and federal eligibility criteria have been on functional handicap and associated cognitive impairment and their behavioural disturb- ances. But at the State level, the Medicaid programme eligibility criteria are still burdened with medical and related criteria which reflect the original assumptive worlds of the mid-seventies (O'Keefe, 1996).

5 A study of Medicaid eligibility criteria in American states illustrates the impact of these older ideas about means and ends (O'Keefe, 1996). Whereas criteria in recent federal proposals have been dominated by capacity to perform essential activities of daily living, the state Medicaid programmes add others whose origins lie in the history of long-term care as an outgrowth of medical services. The patterns are discussed in Davies and Fernández (1997).

the basis of qualifying criteria of a degree of sophistication which matches field decision-making. The more sophisticated attempts to define targeting norms from the actual practice judgements of field-level allocation illustrate that a substantial number of functioning characteristics must be combined in quite complex ways, if decision algorithms are to capture the essence of judgement patterns (see, for instance, a study in Alberta by Coopers and Lybrand, 1994). Though recent American findings show how different are the natural history of need for social care for persons with different diseases (De Lew et al., 1992; Manton and Stallard, 1992; Schauffler et al., 1992), functioning varies greatly for persons with the same disease. So also do the social, psychological and environmental contexts which influence functioning, but the coverage of these is more variable in instrumentation.

Failure to perform essential activities of daily living at home is the most important but not the only need-related dimension which determines the response of workers able and willing to exercise some discretion. However, possible ways of coping and supply influences are also key. So the types of element in assessment instrumentation which best predict allocations are therefore those which use the key information about functional deficits and supply assumptions.

An example is the Isaacs and Neville (1975) classification of users by their 'interval needs'. Based on the assessment in the social and material environment, it requires a judgement based on assumptions about how service interventions can cope with the greatest effect. That is, it requires assumptions about how service inputs can be delivered.

There are several such assumptions. First, there is an implicit assumption that the service personnel will be able to undertake what arises in the time they make themselves available. A second assumption is that there is a correlation between how much input is required and how often attention is required to achieve outcomes most effectively, so that implications for variations in inputs may be crudely described by the frequency with which inputs must take place. Given these assumptions, it is logical that the interval need classification summarises the level of need of a user by the frequency of intervention: more frequently than once a day and at irregular and unpredictable intervals (critical interval need); predictably but once a day (short interval need); and predictably and less frequently (long interval need).

The classification combines both judgements about the key dimensions of need-related circumstances and assumptions about the tasks which the services available perform. Therefore, it is likely that the Isaacs and Neville classification would predict allocations better than a crude classification based on the need-related circumstances (including functional incapacities) by themselves. Some evidence confirms the greater predictive power of the interval needs typology (Davies and Challis, 1986; Davies et al., 1990). Either the classification or a combination of need-related circumstances would predict better than the information in instruments which still reflect origins in health-related services with different conceptions of ends and means: for example, the INSERM instrument used later in this study.

Financing

The financing mechanisms have not been designed to provide the incentives required for home care to fulfil a role mainly of reducing the need to seek places in institutions. One feature is that the system of financing of home care is based on employment with each pension fund. Each pension fund has its own budget, and hence its own criteria of eligibility.[6]

A second aspect is that recent policy argument has added to the goal of allowing persons to be provided with care at home, the aim of creating employment for disadvantaged groups at the edge of society: the creation of *emplois de proximité* as part of the *lutte contre l'exclusion.* The tax concessions available to stimulate such direct employment by users or employment of the potentially *exclus* certainly provide incentives. But the incentives are not finely tailored to combine both effective and efficient use of public funds to support elderly people at high risk of admission to institutions for long-term care, and with effective and efficient generation of jobs among the most marginalised. Policy has been tilted towards the payment of tax allowances for the elderly for the direct employment of private help.

Were the price per hour of such employees to be lower, the number of hours purchased might be greater and the total number in

6 Guillemard and Frossard (1993, p.271) ask: 'Should benefits carry no restrictions? Or should beneficiaries prove they have purchased certain services? Should payments be made to individuals or to a coordinating service (like the case management system in Kent, England)?'

employment might be increased. Both effects are compatible with achieving both policy goals better. This is a discussion which has parallels in other countries: discussions about direct payments in contemporary UK, consumer-directed models in the USA, and in the labour market analyses in the evaluation of the introduction of the Austrian attendance allowances.

Both the Schopflin report of 1991 and the reports on the CNAVTS projects of 1995 clearly favoured service provision rather than cash allowances. They were thought to be the most efficient way of meeting the aim of improving domiciliary care, although no reasons for this belief are actually given. The Chirac proposals for a *chèque autonomie* was a voucher providing consumer choice like an income, but only between alternative methods of procuring care, because the *chèque* was to be exchanged for services although it could be paid to a member of the family or others within or outwith the social circle. But the arrangement created an incentive to reduce the utilisation of formal services. The reason was that it was not accumulable with existing social care entitlements, so that its value against a home help at a standard rate of around 80FF per hour was clearly less than for a private helper who need only receive the SMIC (national minimum wage), which even with social charges only amounts to some 57FF per hour.

Therefore the questions which seem the most fundamental in the French debate on domiciliary care are:

• What is the real effect of the *obligation alimentaire,* and does it favour home rather than residential care?

• Whether, and to what degree, should there remain an incentive to utilise formal agency services? The Schopflin report and arguments put forward by the CNAV were in favour of unified services of the home help and home nursing type, or the payment of cash allowances. But the government seem not to accept that view, judging from fiscal policies and the new arrangement discussed below.

• What are the criteria against which improvements in home care should be judged? Much reform argument such as that in the Schopflin report focus on improving quality and flexibility of response, but these are difficult to measure. What scope for improvements would be revealed were the substitution of home for residential care to become a priority policy objective?

3. Reform proposals

There are perhaps three phases discernible in the recent evolution of French policy reforms since the accession of Chirac to the Presidency. The focus of the first, inherited from the final period of the previous administration, was the *prestation experimentale dépendance* , initiated by the CNAV. During the second, the focus was the Chirac government's initial proposals, the *prestation autonomie dépendance*. During the third, the focus was the allowance which finally passed into law at the end of 1996, the *prestation spécifique dépendance*. These three allowances have significant differences in their content and application, and so merit separate examination. They are summarised in Box 2.

3.1. Prestation expérimentale dépendance (PED)

At the end of 1994, the CNAV launched a new allowance for dependent elderly people, *prestation experimentale dépendance* (PED); it was implemented in twelve project sites from January 1995.[7] It was used to fund services, and only rarely paid as a cash allowance. Its basis was to be the existing *allocation compensatrice pour tierce personne* (ACTP), topped up to the full amount of the new PED, by a *prestation supplementaire dépendance,* for those who would normally only qualify for a percentage of the ACTP. The ACTP element was financed by the *conseils généraux* as part of the *action sociale* budget of the *départements.* The new supplementary payment, the PSD, came from the *caisses de retraite* and was to be financed from their *action sociale* budgets.

The main features were that it would:

- Offer a single referral point for home care.

7 Chirac's new *Ministre de la solidarité entre les générations* conducted consultations with the *partenaires sociaux* and the *conseils généraux* about the *allocation dépendance* from 20 June with a view to its introduction from the end of the year. The *Actualités sociales hebdomadaire* (no. 1932, 23 June 1995) commented: *'Si le débat entre prestations en espèces et prestations en nature n'est pas tranché, le gouvernement tend néanmoins vers une prestation en nature qui éviterait le risque de "thésaurisation". Pour pallier ce risque, il est également envisagé de créer un "chèque autonomie" qui rendrait la "dépense effective"'*. That is confirmed in Bezat (1995).

Box 2. A summary of French proposals for direct payments

- *Allocation compensatrice pour tierce personne* (ACTP), which dates from the *loi de 1975* and is paid by the local authorities through the *aide sociale* budget of the *départements*. It was intended as a payment to disabled adults, but no upper age limit was set for recipients, which has meant that increasingly many *départements* use it as a way of paying for home care for dependent elderly people. It is paid in cash; the upper limit is set nationally as the *majoration pour tierce personne* (MPTP) but the actual percentage allocated to each applicant is decided by the départemental *Commission technique d'orientation et de reclassement professionel* (COTOREP). It is means-tested and liable to be repaid from the recipient's estate.
- *Allocation autonomie et dépendance* (*AAD*), which dates from the days of the Socialist government. See the report by Boulard (Assemblé nationale, 1991) and the report by the Commissariat du plan (Schopflin, 1991). The actual legislative framework for the AAD passed through the Chamber of Deputies in March 1993, but was abandoned with the fall of the Bérégovoy administration at the end of that year. It was modelled on the ACTP formula of a cash payment administered through the *départements* using a revised version of the COTOREP to be called a *Commission départemental d'évaluation de la dépendance*. The extra cost to the *départements* was to be met from national expenditure in the form of equalisation payments, the total cost of which was estimated to be 1 millard FF.
- *Prestation éxperimentale dépendance* (PED). Introduced by the Caisse national d'assurance vieillesse des travailleurs salariés (CNAVTS) at the start of 1995 in twelve trial *départements*. It consists of the existing ACTP paid by the *département* through *aide sociale*, topped up to a higher level by a *prestation supplementaire dépendance* (PSD), funded from the existing *action sociale* budgets of CNAVTS and other major existing funders of standard domiciliary care. It is paid in kind, either directly to the service supply agency, or by means of the voucher system, *chèque service*. Assessment is by multidisciplinary teams using a standard scale, AGGIR, attribution being made by the COTOREP.

Box 2. Continued

- *Prestation d'autonomie dépendance* (PAD). The initial proposals during the early stages of Chirac's presidency, introduced by Prime Minister Balladur in 1995. It was intended to be a more generous allowance than ACTP and, unlike the PED, it would be controlled exclusively by the *départements* and would be paid to recipients of both domiciliary and institutional care. Like the PED, it would be paid in kind, using the same assessment procedures and using a similar voucher system, the *chèque autonomie*. It was dropped in July 1996 as being currently too expensive to introduce.
- *Préstation spécifique dépendance* (PSD). The less ambitious proposals evolved from the PAD, which eventually passed into law under Prime Minister Juppé in early 1997. They are just coming into effect at the time of writing. It is to be an allowance paid in kind and using the *chèque service* voucher system but, although there is a national maximum, the actual level payable is fixed by each *département*. It cannot be added to any other home care benefit such as *aide ménagère*, and there are plans to extend its payment to those in institutional care as well as at home.

• Provide a holistic assessment of the applicant's home care needs. This would be undertaken by a multidisciplinary team of both general medical doctors and social workers. The doctors and social workers would be employees of any of the collaborating *caisses* or the *département*.

• Offer a locality-based approach by the assessment teams to facilitate the interweaving of formal and informal resources, and to facilitate continuity of responsibility for the ongoing care management.

• Establish a contractual care plan, once the needs assessment had been agreed by the assessment team, the elderly person and their informal carers.

In total, 41 *départements* offered to act as hosts for the pilot project and, of these, twelve were chosen because they were likely to be able to improve on already good working relationships between the partner

Box 3. The Ille et Vilaine project

The argument and arrangements for one of the twelve project areas, Ille et Vilaine (35), drew heavily on the Kent Community Care Project model of budget-holding case management. This was separately evaluated by the Ecole nationale de la santé publique (ENSP). Finance and fieldwork staff were contributed by the *département*, the CNAV, through its regional office, CRAM de Bretagne, and other main funders of care, such as the *mutualité sociale agricole* (MSA).

The care management role was undertaken by joint teams of locality-based social workers and general medical doctors, drawn from the partner agencies. The allowance, once agreed, financed the implementation of an individual care plan, tailored closely to the user's need-related circumstances. Help was provided by normal service supply associations, newer *associations mandataire*, and by directly employed neighbours or others mobilised on a case-specific basis. Caseload levels dictated that the monitoring and review functions of case management be delegated to a key worker in each case, whether the service supply association, a family member, or the user themselves.

The ENSP report on the project at the end of its first full year highlighted several points which reflect findings from the British experience both of the initial budget-holding case management projects and also subsequently with the generalisation post-1993.

- *Competition.* The effect of the competition generated by the PED led to previously monopolistic services having to improve their availability and quality, with the user now having a central role as employer, and will also lead to the development of a private, for profit sector.
- *Implementation period.* The first two years were seen as a period of *apprentissage*, when the new techniques were being learnt and the experiences digested.

agencies. From the outset, it was intended that there should be a national evaluation of the allowance. It was to focus on:

Box 3. Continued

- *Innovation by example.* While the British examples of budget-holding case management have not seen ready replication since the generalisation of the reforms, they were seen as an outcome in the Ille et Vilaine project, where the collaborative working engendered was felt to have had a wider influence in the activities of partner organisations. The problem of transplanting the project to other *départements* where there were not the pre-existing conditions such as a similar social policy for the elderly run by sufficiently experienced staff was highlighted, again something which has echoes in the UK.
- *Service effects.* Some traditional and long-established services clearly had difficulty in adapting to a more user-centred approach, failing to offer flexible responses to need; others which acted as a single point of contact for the user would react creatively by looking outside their normal staff to meet specific need; finally, new organisations set up recently, such as the *association mandataire,* offered a more responsive and flexible approach.
- *Care management implications.* The ENSP report quotes an assessment time of between 6.5 and 8 hours, and around a further 20 hours for the completion of the setting-up period because of the complexity of care packaging. This has similarities with the UK experience, and emphasises the time-consuming nature of the care management process.
- *Effect on informal care.* The report notes the finding that often the payment of one family member for their caring role could lead to other members of the family withdrawing. This is of interest in the UK with the debate here on the introduction of direct payments.

- The mobilisation of the various agencies involved in the area of the dependent elderly. This theme recurs in French argument and local initiatives.
- The impacts of the new allocation on costs and financial transfers.

• Validation of the new *grille de dépendance* (AGGIR). The intention was that it should be universally applied by all institutions.

• Coordination at the level of the individual and the family, in order to provide one single point of contact.

• Coordination of the offer and management of the new allocation.

It was stated that the establishment of the projects was not to be taken to imply the creation of a new allocation, but it was expected that it would result in a new national allowance two years subsequently. Part of the CNAV's agenda may also have been to attempt to capture the initiative in the developing struggle for control of the eventual national allowance. The competing claims seem to be those of the *conseils généraux* in the *départements*, which eventually proved to be the case.

The national evaluation of the PED was undertaken by CNAV and Centre de recherche pour l'étude et l'observation des conditions de vie (CREDOC) during a period of one year. Their report was submitted to the Assemblée des présidents de conseils généraux (APCG) in the autumn of 1996 (Simon, 1997). The overall conclusion was that the experiment 'could be considered generally as successful', with several good points: good coordination between the respective agencies involved, coherent assessment, the mobilisation and coordination of services at the level of the individual user, improved recognition of the needs of informal carers and the development of multidisciplinary working (*Actualités sociales hebdomadaire*, no. 1996, 8 November 1996). But there were difficulties. For instance, there was a large increase in workload, and it was the difficult to achieve successful assessments within the expected time limits. These implied a need to simplify procedures. It was also argued that the AGGIR assessment scale should be made more supple, and should cover a wider range of need-related circumstances.

It was estimated that there would be 200,000 beneficiaries, compared with the 500,000 estimated to benefit from the earlier aborted *prestation dépendance autonomie* (Simon, 1997, p.1).

The Ille et Vilaine Care Management Project

PSSRU's connection with the Ille et Vilaine was direct. Among the persons visiting were the director of CRAM de Bretagne and senior officials of its social work department, followed through by PSSRU presentations to CNAV's *service d'action sociale* at Paris, and to a conference organised by CRAM de Bretagne at Quiberon (see Box 3).

The Schopflin report in 1991 discussed the Kent Community Care Project model of case management for the elderly[8] in its account of the relevance to France of systems in other countries (Commissariat général du plan, 1991, p.90). Papers about that project had been published in France from the early eighties (Challis and Davies, 1981; Davies, 1981). Parties of French agency managers and senior professionals, including senior officials from agencies in Ille et Vilaine, had made structured observation visits to Kent annually since 1988, hosted by PSSRU; PSSRU personnel also made visits to CRAM de Brétagne. Therefore it was not surprising that one of the models for the trial areas involved in the PED was strongly influenced by the Kent Community Care Project.

The project drew together the *département*, who were already responsible for the ACTP allowance, and the other major funders of home care for the elderly, particularly CRAM and MSA. The fieldwork was the responsibility of area-based, multidisciplinary teams. The partner organisations pooled their home care budgets through the COTOREP, an organisation at the level of the *département*.

The multidisciplinary teams performed the care management roles of assessment, care planning, coordination, innovation, review and re-assessment, with the work of case finding being undertaken by either the local *Centre communal d'action sociale* (CCAS), or similar structures within the other partners to the project. Once the individual budget had been determined by the COTOREP, assessment and care planning was undertaken at the level of the agency. The budget was spent on a care plan formally agreed between the care management team, the user and their informal carers.

The field teams had a total of 42 *équipes medico-sociale*, field staff drawn from the partner agencies: 18 social workers from CRAM, 11 from the *conseil général* and 13 from MSA, together with 8 doctors from CRAM and the *conseil général*. The care management teams dealt with 2,700 cases in a full year, of which 1,419 were accepted for receipt of

---

8 *La nécessité d'un arbitrage entre les bénéficiares potentiels est clairement posée et c'est à l'autorité locale de l'effectuer. Dans le cas où le financement public est conséquent, il faut nommer un gestionnaire de cas, 'case manager', qui assure de la bonne allocation de ressources et de l'efficacité de l'action menée* (Schopflin, 1991, p.90).

the PED. Of these users, 51 per cent, the PED was greater than the equivalent allowance paid under the normal ACTP arrangements.

The time-consuming nature of the care management process, in part due to the need to use the national assessment scale, AGGIR, often led the care management teams to delegate the monitoring part of their function to a case-specific person or agency. But the overall case responsibility remained with the teams to ensure continuity of care. The delegation of the budget, as in the KCCP, to the level of the workers at user level allowed much resourcefulness to be shown in making use of the user's existing informal care network, and in paying client-specific helpers, for example neighbours or family members. Of time contributed, 38 per cent was from directly employed helpers, 31 per cent from helpers employed through the *association mandataire*, 22 per cent from family members, and only 9 per cent from traditional home help associations. The evaluators reported that the use of this new allowance caused the traditional services to adapt their response to the needs of the individual. For example, they increased their availability at weekends or evenings.

The average response time between application and initial setting-up of the care plan was similar to that in the UK's post-reform care management in England and Wales (Davies et al., 1997). The problem of the time-consuming nature of budget-holding case management emphasises the need for targeting of the care management function.

The overall reaction — of the *département*, CRAM, field workers and users — was positive.

3.2. *Prestation autonomie dépendance (PAD)*

One basic conclusion of the initial four months of the new *prestation dépendance* (PED) during Balladur's government was unsurprising: the assessment process was time-consuming. Care management was itself a resource which required careful targeting. There remained fundamental technical problems still to be solved. One was whether vouchers were to be provided via the *chèque service* system, or whether there was to be an entitlement to services from a chosen agency. There was a rising tide of government unpopularity in the public opinion polls. Countries in the European Community were starting the long struggle to meet the requirements of the Maastricht Treaty for members of the group allowed to adopt the common European currency. The new Chirac régime, under Prime Minister Juppé, announced its proposals for the *prestation dépendance* in mid-September 1995. They were to come into effect from 1 January 1996 for those elderly recipients living in the community, and the following 1 January 1997 for those in institutional care. At the end of 1995, following the widespread social unrest and continued uncertainty over the balancing of the social security budgets, the introduction of the *prestation autonomie* was again deferred. It was to be introduced in a less ambitious form from 1 January 1997.

Probably the two major features of the new allowance were that it was to be controlled by the *conseils généraux* (thus outflanking the initiative by the CNAV), no doubt reflecting political pressure from the Sénat whose members exert significant influence on the local politicians of the *départements,* and that the allowance would be paid as an entitlement, provided direct to the recipient using the device of the *chèque service* (see Glossary). The effect of the latter would be to reduce the influence of the *associations,* who of course were direct recipients of the existing home care funding for *aide menagère, garde à domicile* and *soins à domicile.*

Assessment and functional dependence

To obtain the allowance, the person would have to undergo a dependency assessment. The assessment would be undertaken by multidisciplinary teams, of which one member had to be a doctor, the other two or more members being perhaps a psychologist, social worker or representative from the CNAV or other *caisses.* This dependency assessment was to be based on the AGGIR scale. The implementation of this had been evaluated in some *départements* during the previous two years or more (see Box 4). It made assessment criteria more explicit than the general ACTP assessment. However, it was criticised by the *Conseil économique et social* (CES) for not taking into account all of the social circumstances of the applicant (*Actualités sociales hebdomadaire,* 1996). In particular, it took no account of the inputs of informal carers, still less of these carers' own needs. Certainly it did not include psychological factors such as the users' motivation, nor relational aspects of the users' informal care networks. This is perhaps not surprising, since it was in fact designed as a means of assessing individuals as an aid to care

Box 4. AGGIR assessment scale

The seventeen points covered in the assessment are each rated on a three-point scale, as follows:

A Can regularly perform the task unaided and normally correctly.
B Can partially perform the task.
C Cannot perform the task.

1 Coherence: can conduct a coherent conversation.
2 Orientation: aware of time, period of the day, place.
3 Washing: personal care.
4 Dressing: can dress/undress.
5 Feeding: can manage prepared meals.
6 Toileting: can manage bodily functions.
7 Transfers: can get up, get to bed, sit in a chair.
8 Mobility: within the house, with or without stick, frame or wheelchair.
9 Mobility: outside, not including use of means of transport.
10 Communication: can use telephone, alarm call systems, etc.
11 Finances: can manage own finances, budget, possessions.
12 Meals: can prepare and serve meals.
13 Housework: can do housework tasks.
14 Transport: can use means of transport.
15 Shopping: can shop, directly or by correspondence.
16 Medication: can follow instructions given by the doctor.
17 Hobbies: can undertake leisure activities, sporting, social or cultural.

Source: Computer disk AGGIR W v.2, *An Iso Resource Group computing program*, National Syndicate of Clinical Gerontology, Centre Hospitalier, Le Mans.

planning, not to deducing eligibility for a cash allowance, even less on the need to enter shelter-with-care. Its attraction to the Government was that it was computerisable and it reduced a range of variables to a six-point score, Groupe Iso-ressource (GIR) 1 to 6.

As an example of the difficulty in making fine judgements when using the AGGIR *grille* one can cite an exercise conducted by the authors, using the *grille* for three theoretical cases where only the variable for help with transfer to or from a bed or chair was altered. If the assessment was made on the basis of being independent for this task, the GIR level was 5, if partially dependent the level was GIR 4, and if fully dependent GIR 2.

Income test and récuperation sur succession
In addition to this assessment of dependency, there was also a financial assessment, with an upper income limit of 13,000FF per month or, excluding any income from the new allowance, 9,250FF per month. Any money paid under this allowance was not to be subject to the *obligation alimentaire*, but, like ACTP, was subject to a charge on the inheritance after the death of the recipient. In the official press release following the announcement of the new allowance, an example was given which showed how the new allowance compared to the existing ACTP (see Box 5).

Box 5. ACTP/Prestation d'autonomie for a given income

	Allocation compensatrice (ACTP)	Prestation d'autonomie
Gross income	6,500FF	6,500FF
Net income	4,680FF	4,680FF
Amount payable	4,300FF	4,300FF
Total income	8,980FF	8,980FF
Income limit	7,600FF	9,250FF
Reduction due to income limit	1,380FF	Nil
Amount payable	2,920FF	4,300FF

Monitoring the use of the benefit
The allocation payable was to be given to the recipient in the form of a *chèque autonomie*, to be modelled on the existing *chèque service*, and processed through the same government department, URSSAF, which also deals with the social security payments under the present system. There was also to be a system to provide for returns from the URSSAF to *départements* so that they could monitor who actually received the

payments financed by the new allowance. This was intended to reduce the alleged misuse of the ACTP cash allowance. The allowance could not now simply be added to the recipient's savings account or tucked away under the mattress. Also, monitoring would ensure that the payments were actually going to the intended carer. However, up to 10 per cent of the allowance could be paid in cash specifically for personal care supplies. Spouses were specifically excluded from receiving the allowance, but other members of the family who provided care could be paid, as with private employed helpers or, if the help was provided by an *association*, they were to be reimbursed directly by the *département*.

Cost to public funds

The *départemental* expenditure on care of the elderly is 9 billion FF per annum, of which 6 billion are for *aide sociale* and the other 3 billion for ACTP (Schopflin, 1991, p.33).

For the first year, the new allowance would have been likely to cost 14 billion FF, the shortfall having to be made good by central government from the Fonds national de solidarité vieillesse.[9] On the assumption that the allowance would be extended to those in residential care, originally intended from 1997, the full-year cost was estimated to rise to 20 billion FF.

3.3. *Prestation spécifique dépendance* (PSD)

The increasing financial constraints on the French Government led the Prime Minister, M. Juppé to announce on the 5 July 1996 that although the planned *prestation autonomie* would not be 'buried', it would be intro-

9 The shortfall in the Fonds was in part to be financed by increased taxes such as the *contribution sociale généralisé* (CSG), which is applied across all income, particularly pension income which had enjoyed a favourable income tax régime. In part it was to be financed by increased taxes on wines and spirits and then, in 1996, by the *remboursement de la dette sociale* (RDS), an even more widely-drawn tax intended to cover the existing deficit in the social security funds. The new Socialist government of M. Jospin, in its first budget, proposed an even greater switch of social costs, particularly health, to these more generally drawn funds (*Le Monde*, 18 Sept 1997).

duced in a more limited version than originally planned. The following week, a bill was introduced for a *prestation spécifique dépendance*.

The goal of the PSD was more limited. It aimed to extend the existing ACTP, but with the use of the AGGIR scale to provide a national basis for the assessment process. The allowance was to have lower budget caps and income ceilings, the maximum budget cap being just above the basic ACTP, 5,596FF per month. In practice, this would be payable at an upper limit of 80 per cent of this amount, and the upper income limit was set at 10,477FF per month, compared with the original proposal of 9,239FF per month.

Unlike the PED, the allowance would be allocated to those in institutional care as well as at home. The payment would be linked to the level of dependency of the recipient rather than the category of institution. The allowance as originally proposed would be available to persons of lower levels of dependency for those in some form of shelter-with-care (AGGIR scales 1-5, against 1-3 for those applicants in the community). This itself would have tended to generate further problems, both for the shelter-with-care providers who aim at a mix of lower and higher dependency clients within one housing unit, and for those elderly people who are at the lowest level of income.

For the care home providers, there is now a debate as to whether they should provide their own arms' length home care organisations of the *mandataire* type, in order to access the PSD paid to their residents and so focus their efforts on a more nursing home level of clients, or whether to look to a wider diversification into resource centres for the local community, perhaps with home care services operating a day centre and a telephone-based alarm call system. This would enable the mix of care home clients to remain the same, with more active residents being in effect cross-subsidised by the opening out of services to dependent elderly people wishing to remain in their own homes. But for those users at home who are in the lower dependency categories, and so unable to qualify for the new allowance, there would have been a perverse incentive to enter a care home and so qualify for the PSD payable to dependency levels 4 and 5, and thus unsurprisingly this proposal was soon dropped, the allowance only being paid to those in GIR 1 to 3, regardless of their place of residence.

Such is the complexity of the change from paying people according to their level of dependency rather than the category of care home in which they live, however, that the date for the introduction of this stage of the PSD reforms, linked to general reform of the tariffication of shelter-with-care provision, is not currently scheduled until mid-1998. The present tariffication rests upon the category of the home, either residential, medicalised or hospital sector, and divides the daily charge into two sections: basic costs — the *prix de journée*, payable by the resident, their family or *départemental aide sociale*; and the medical care costs — *cure médicale* payable by CNAM.

The new tariffication will represent a significant change in that for the first time in France, medical provision, such as the hospital *moyen* and *long séjour* beds will now be subject, at least in part, to social rather than health legislation. Each care home will need to negotiate precise agreements between the home, the local authority and the health authority over who pays for which aspect of the overall medical, board and lodging and social care costs and a new factor, the cost element attributable to dependency. It will also put the *conseil généraux* in a key position to control planning for places in all categories of shelter-with-care provision, since it can control directly the payment of the dependency element, even to long-stay patients in hospital beds.

The new PSD brought no new money to finance the care of the elderly, but it did at least restore the ACTP to its original function. The ACTP had been intended as an allowance for younger physically handicapped adults rather than for dependent older people. In many local authorities, therefore, it is likely that little will change, except that it will mean extra expense for local authorities, already beginning to count the financial cost of the increasing decentralisation of government functions, and who now have to provide a multidisciplinary assessment and extend their previously limited application of ACTP. In fact, although the new allowance has a statutory upper limit, each *département* has the authority to fix its level up to that limit. Thus some, such as the Hauts de Seine (92), a wealthier Paris suburb, have set it at 4,400FF per month, whereas some hard-pressed rural *départements*, such as the Corrèze (19), have set the allowance at only 1,140FF per month. For those *conseils généraux* who pursue a more innovative developmental policy towards the care of the elderly, the new legislation could encourage the development of jointly-financed, multidisciplinary budget-holding case management schemes, but not under as favourable conditions as those promised by the earlier experimental allowance

(PED). Of course, those currently operating the PED will have to revert to the new, lower allowance for all new applicants, and current recipients will come within its terms at the next annual review of their situation.

The new allowance not only fails to pull together funding from various agencies in the way that the *prestation expérimentale dépendance* was designed to do, but also it does not introduce any other new government funding. It also explicitly forbids its accumulation with existing home care provision. In one *département* for which we have evidence, the average level of ACTP received, after assessment for dependency and income, is about 1,900FF per month,[10] this would finance only about 24 hours per month of *aide ménagère*, less than the standard CNAV allocation. The degree of shortfall is highlighted by the average figure of top-up granted by the PED, of 1,225.63FF per month for the same *département*. Because domiciliary recipients will have to use the allowance to pay for direct service provision, there will be an increased incentive to choose and develop support at lower costs using, for instance, the brokerage organisation, *associations mandataire*, or direct employment by users using the *chèque service*. In this latter case, spouses could not be paid by this allowance. But as we shall show below, the exclusion of spouses need not prevent the money remaining within the family, so much of it might not be directly used to create fresh employment of others.[11]

Role of the départements

The current reforms in France will make the system there more similar to that in the UK. The Griffiths report confirmed and reinforced the position of the major local authorities as the local agencies responsible for financing, commissioning market development and regulation. The new reforms in France give the main role to the *départements*, the local

---

10 The Direction de la Prevention et de l'Action Social Committee paper of the Département de l'Ain, December 1996, quotes an average ACTP figure of 1,889.27FF.

11 One conclusion in the ENSP report on the Ille et Vilaine project (Jourdin, 1996, p.21) was that one full-time equivalent post at the level of the minimum wage (SMIC) would be created for every three recipients of the PED. However, this was calculated theoretically and did not differentiate between family and non-family paid helpers.

government tier most closely resembling the county councils who have the key role in the British reforms.

The *conseils généraux* of the *départements* are responsible for managing the new allowance, setting in place the multidisciplinary teams, integrating their work with the other agencies such as the *caisses*, ensuring the development of an overall *départemental* plan (the *plan gérontologique départemental*), and ensuring that recipients and their families, through the multidisciplinary teams, receive case management inputs such as needs assessments, care planning advice, and evaluation of effectiveness and quality. Described thus, the range and nature of the tasks seem strikingly similar to those in the post-reform UK.

To meet criticism from such national agencies as the CNAV that, under the management of the *départements*, the implementation will vary excessively across the country, the government has proposed a monitoring body, the Observatoire de la dépendance. It will be within the remit of the Ministre de la solidarité entre les génerations. On it will be represented the *caisses*, the *départements* and organisations for the elderly.

Concerns

The proposals have caused concern among the main service supply *associations*. The concerns have been partly met by the government in that they have required that only those agencies who are agreed service suppliers can be contracted by *départements*. Private, for-profit organisations[12] have been specifically excluded. In addition, the *associations* have been granted fiscal parity with directly employed domiciliary helps in that, for the 1996 tax year, a deduction of 50 per cent of the cost of charges for home care up to a maximum of 90,000FF can be allowed against the total tax due from an individual recipient.

There are hints of further difficulties to come. For instance, one of the smaller *caisses*, *caisse de retraite des ouvriers de bâtiment*, has indicated

12 It is interesting to note that a combination of major private firms such as SODEXHO, a principal catering contractor to the shelter-with-care sector, together with the Caisse des Dépôts, a quasi-governmental finance house, joined together to form the Société de développement pour l'emploi dans les services (SDES), which is now actively canvassing its services as a private, for-profit supplier of domiciliary care (SDES letter to FASSAD, 16 December 1996).

that, from 1 July 1997, it will no longer pay for home help for its pensioners. This will result in the withdrawal of service from lower dependency clients, higher dependency clients being able to subsidise the cost of home care by the PSD. At present this is just an isolated example of the complete withdrawal of pension funds from the use of their *action sociale* budgets to finance home care. However, the recent CNAV Circulaire 51/97 of 13 June 1997 makes clear that this major financer of domiciliary care will no longer pay for home help for its pensioners if they are eligible for the new PSD — that is, are in AGGIR dependency ranges 1 to 3 — even if they choose not to apply for the allowance, although it will still finance intensive, short-term personal care by means of *garde à domicile*, for example for up to six months on discharge from hospital.[13] Thus, taken in conjunction with (i) the financial incentive to those receiving the allowance to purchase care direct or by means of a brokerage service, and (ii) the emergence of the private, for-profit sector in home care, the position of the traditional suppliers is challenged.

The traditional home care *associations* feel threatened by the impartiality of the reforms. It is perhaps indicative of the complexity of the effects which this allowance will create for all *départements*, for home care and shelter-with-care providers, that although the main legislation was passed in January 1997, the detailed implementing regulations were not published in the *Journal officiel* until 28 April 1997, to come into force from 1 June 1997 for those at home, and not until some later date the

13 The likely outcomes from this *circulaire* will show wide regional variations in its interpretation. While there are indications that some *caisses régionale d'assurance maladie* (CRAM) will take a strict approach, only offering domiciliary care to those of their pension recipients who are in the lower categories of dependency (GIR 4 to 6), others, notably that for the Ile de France (CRAMIF), will offer services to those not only in the lower dependency, but also to those in the higher GIR 1 to 3 categories who would otherwise have qualified for the new PSD but for their income being higher than the maximum permitted under the PSD regulations. In addition, CRAMIF is planning to introduce a care-managed response. All applicants for home care will have an assessment from one of their social work staff, who will draw up a care plan and, if the CRAMIF does not have a contract with a suitable service provider, will undertake the liaison required with other agencies, such as the Centre communal d'action social (CCAS) to ensure implementation of the care plan.

following year for those in institutional care, probably the end of August 1998.

Criticism of the proposals to date depends on the perspective and interests of the commentator.

• CNAV expresses the view that the decentralisation of the administration of the new allowance to the *conseils généraux* risks excessive variability across the country. The wide range in the actual maxima of the PSD between *départements* and the difference in treatment of persons at the margin of dependency to qualify for the PSD or standard home help provision only serve to emphasise the justice of this view.

• Service supply agencies would have preferred it to have been mandatory for the allowance to be paid directly to themselves, as with present home help funding since, they argue, this would ensure that home care staff employed by the new money will be adequately trained and supported: an argument which seems less than convincing in the light of British experiences of amateurism and idiosyncrasy in assessment processes and outcomes. (The government had indicated that they expected this new arrangement to create 50,000 new jobs.) Service supply agencies argue that these jobs will simply be directly employed and untrained workers, replacing existing home care staff but on lower wages.

• Some social care organisations providing institutional care criticise the allowance for failing to meet the promised shortfall in funding for medicalised care beds;[14] and some for distorting the balance of potential residents through the linking of the allowance to the individual rather than the category of home.[15]

• All the interest groups argue that the allowance will be insufficient to meet the needs of the highest cost users. This is probably valid. The allowance is not added to any existing home help entitlement, but is intended to stand alone in funding the social care package required.

---

14 The Minister responsible for the new allowance, M. Barrot, has been quoted as accepting that 14,000 medical care beds and 4,000 home nursing care places, which have already been agreed in previous years' budgets, have still not been created (*Les Dossiers de l'ADEPHA*, 1997).

15 In one exercise reported to the authors, a local authority home with 50 per cent of its beds classified as medicalised found that over 60 per cent of its residents were at levels of dependency sufficient to qualify for the PSD (GIR 1-3).

Assuming (i) that the recipients of the proposed new allocation will be similar to those qualifying for the existing ACTP; (ii) that, using a finding reported below, 80.5 per cent of such cases had a member of the family other than the spouse in addition to, or exclusively, acting as an informal carer; and (iii) that the family would prefer to retain the allowance rather than spend it outside the family to buy in care from an agency, the new allowance would generate new employment in only a relatively small proportion of cases. If the allowance furthermore replaces existing entitlement to home help, the scope for real employment creation seems further reduced. The redistribution of income to relatives will far exceed the payments corresponding to new care inputs from informal and quasi-informal providers.

So the new allowance, PSD, falls far short of the interim PED, let alone the Chirac government's original aims as expressed in the *allocation autonomie*. But, as is claimed by the Ministre at the time of its introduction, it is *'un lifting de l'ACTP'* (Barrot, *Ministre du travail et des affaires sociales*) and it is intended that it will be an interim measure only: *'une prestation de transition qui devra être améliorée dès que la situation financière de la France sera plus saine'* (Rousseau, 1997). Since the administration of Lionel Jospin came to power, the new Health Minister, Mme Aubry, has been noticeably silent on the issue of the PSD, but political pressure, not only from service providers of home and residential care but also from the unions speaking on behalf of pensioners, is growing for a review of the current provision and even for it to be financed via the national *sécurité social* budget rather than left to *départements*.[16]

Timing is vital in the history of social reform. In the UK, the Attlee government created the welfare state by nationalisation and the consolidation of power while the UK still enjoyed a temporary economic advantage, and before it was understood how devastating would be the relative decline of the four subsequent decades in national competitiveness compared with European neighbours. The inter-war structures in the UK were more like those maintained post-war in France. Such optimism was impossible. The new ambitions conceived during the early optimism of the first Wilson administration of the

16 *Actualités sociales hebdomadaire*, No. 2038, 26 September 1997. The *Dernières Nouvelles d'Alsace* of 26 November 1997, in an item headlined *Les retraités dans la rue*, reported on public demonstrations by pensioners against, *inter alia*, the variation between *départements* in their application of the new PSD.

sixties were worked through to legislation and consolidated into structures before the Oil Crisis and devaluation halted development. The post-Griffiths reforms were enacted and implemented without the constraints in the French context of an overwhelming policy priority to keep in line with Germany, maintain the franc fort, *assainir le Sécu* and satisfy the Maastricht criteria to join the EMU.

L'amélioration, if not more, will be eagerly awaited. What has been put in place gives the user the chance to tap sources of services other than those provided by the conventional agencies, and so achieve more welfare for the expenditure, even if for-profit providers remain, at least for the present, excluded. In this respect, the system is more consumer-directed than the British. Again, the arrangements focus on the individual assessment and care management arrangements, but the assessment protocol and procedures bias against some need-related circumstances, far less take advantage of second-generation assessment thinking. The focus on a budget level for the individual encourages action to use the resources most equitably and efficiently by introducing a sense of opportunity cost, given the presence of a capped departmental budget. But funding from the various sources has not been pooled, encouraging cost-shunting, the distortion of agency priorities and exacerbating territorial inequity. For the first time, a single allowance is paid whether the recipient is at home or in facilities, whether social or medical. But France has certainly taken some steps towards putting in place some of the preconditions for improving equity and efficiency in its arrangements; and may have created arrangements which will actually contribute greatly to *'le réforme profond du systême'* which the Schopflin report thought to be an essential prerequisite for better targeting.

Part II

4 Study design

1. Collection of evidence

1.1. Research foci

This study contributes to enhancing our knowledge about who gets what where; and how that changes between the initial allocation of services, and the second and third six-monthly reviews. Its focus is around home care services. In particular, it allows the comparison of levels of home care service obtained for persons aged 60 and over of different levels of disability in a number of French and English areas of various kinds: rural, urban and suburban. It also examines the relationship between need-related circumstances and services. For the French sites, it looks at three possible models of response to needs, and at outcomes over time for the applicants.

At core, the aims of the proposed study were (i) to examine the relationship between need-related circumstances and service allocation for new recipients dependent on public funds in each of a number of areas; (ii) to show how the need-related circumstances change among the initial recipients; (iii) to show the proportions for whom further service is requested at the end of the initial period and what services they were allocated; and (iv) to determine the outcomes for those who cease to be recipients of home-based services.

From these data, it has been possible to examine the effect on the probability of admission to institutional care on various need-related circumstances and types and quantities of service inputs, to estimate the scope for improvement in home-based services, and to examine the relative effectiveness of service provision compared with cash allowances in reducing the probability of entry into residential care.

1.2. Data collection

Evidence was collected in three sites in France. For Great Britain, the data were collected from a study undertaken by the PSSRU in 1984, the Domiciliary Care Project. In the wider British study, ten sites provided data on a total of 589 consumers. However, the present study was narrowed where appropriate, to enable cross-country matching of sites by broad area characteristics: suburbs with mixed income groups on the fringe of a capital city; rural areas primarily dependent on agriculture; and medium-sized market towns. The study was restricted to the investigation of recipients of *aide sociale* or other publicly-funded assistance (for example, ACTP, benefits from CNAVTS and similar agencies) and their equivalents in England and Wales. This simplifies and makes less expensive the procedures for obtaining the evidence required. The French sites provided three models of response to the delivery of home care. One gave policy priority for the payment of cash allowances (ACTP) in preference to service provision. Another site was an example of the unified home nursing/home help services endorsed in the Schopflin report. The third implemented a model for the co-ordination of separate home nursing, home help and *garde à domicile*, providing a single point of entry, also endorsed as an aim in the Schopflin and other reports.

The levels of input and dependency characteristics were defined in the form *Demande ACTP* used by one of the French sites, and accepted by the other two sites so as to ensure standardised data. Basically, the information collected includes:

- marital status, household composition and the situation of children not living in the household;
- information about housing and social contacts;
- information about inability to perform tasks of daily living and so on;
- a statement of the needs justifying the application;
- eligibility for *aide sociale* or other public funding through the local authority;
- hours requested and agreed, either as service or as a cash equivalent;
- inputs of informal help and formal help for each task for which assistance is provided; and

• outcomes for those who cease to receive home care and the date at which that occurred.

Similar data were collected at six- and twelve-month intervals so that changes could be described, together with the reasons and date for termination of service if that were the case.

The information collected made it possible to examine the relationship between need-related circumstances, informal help and formal inputs, and to analyse the probability of various inputs and need-related circumstances leading to entry into institutional care.

1.3. Study features

Where required for the statistical modelling, the two countries' databases were matched by other client characteristics, as explained in the relevant chapters.

The French study was based on the British Domiciliary Care Project. The main features of each study are summarised in Box 6. The principal difference is the smaller scale and shorter duration of the French study, and the emphasis in the French study on the estimation of the time given to caregiving tasks from informal as well as formal sources. Levels of dependency were assessed according to the scales shown in Box 7, to enable comparisons to be drawn between countries, and to note the possible value of different measures of dependency as predictors of outcome.

The French sites who participated in the study were Athis Mons, La Manche and St Omer, and the areas and their service delivery characteristics are explained in more detail in Chapter 7. The British sites were from areas with broadly similar social characteristics to the French sites to which they are matched in those tables which give comparative data. The source for the British data is the Domiciliary Care Project. The Domiciliary Care Project convention was that sites were not identified by their proper names. The British Area 1 in this study is a largely rural shire county, Area 2 a metropolitan borough and Area 3 a shire county but with a higher level of industrialisation than Area 1. The larger sample of British users from all the ten areas in the Domiciliary Care Project was drawn upon where appropriate, as noted in the relevant sections of the book.

Box 6. Study features

Focus on needs, resources & outcomes	*England & Wales*	*France*
Statistical descriptions and modelling analysis. Explanation and illumination by studying structures, policies, assumptive worlds, practice and processes. Databases	Interviews with 589 consumers at first referral or at major change in support package. Interviews with 443 of the consumers approximately six months later. Interviews with 210 'principal carers' of the consumers contemporaneously with the second consumer interview. Resources for consumers tracked until death, admission to an institution for long-term care, or second consumer interview. Data from consumers collected over six months from SSD workers most likely to perform care tasks of case management using the case review instrument. Data about relocation, mortality and utilisation after three years. Analysis of SSD and community health service documentation.	Interviews with 198 consumers of publicly-funded domiciliary support at time of first application for a new input. Interviews with 110 of the consumers who were still receiving domiciliary services after approximately six months. Assessment of time devoted to care tasks at time of initial interviews for 153 consumers and then subsequently for the 83 still in the community at the time of the second interviews. Details of formal services inputs collected at time of second and third interviews after six and twelve months, or until death, admission to long-term care or other reason for terminating services. Data from consumers collected by those field workers having direct contact with them as result of the initial application for domiciliary care, and subsequently after six and twelve months. Data about relocation, mortality and utilisation after 18 months. Analysis of Départemental Schema Gérontologique, Annual reports.

Box 6. Continued

Interviews about structures, policy process, practice and assumptive worlds with agency personnel.	e.g. social work team leaders, area officers, SSD headquarters policy-makers, participants in innovatory social services schemes.	e.g. departmental and field level health and social services staff, background material from La Fondation de France, UNIOPSS, Government reports (for example, by Schopflin and Boulard).
Analysis of secondary data bases:	e.g. 1985 General Household Survey, CIPFA and DHSS statistics	e.g. Ministère des Affaires Sociales, CNAVTS

Box 7. Needs categorisations

INSERM need category

Definition

1st group: People confined to bed or armchair

2nd group: People not confined to bed or armchair but needing help from another person for washing and dressing

3rd group: People not confined to bed or armchair or needing help from another person for washing and dressing, but unable to leave their house without help from another person

4th group: Independent people or those dependent for instrumental activities — needing help with domestic tasks

Interval need level

Definition: Isaacs and Neville interval need level

Critical: Bed/chairbound, need help with toileting; incontinent or severe mental problems

Short: Need help with meals/snacks, washing, dressing or getting to bed

Long: Need help with instrumental activities of daily living, such as shopping

Independent: Not needing help with instrumental activities of daily living (IADLs)

POW QI weighted general ADL index

Definition: Production of welfare quasi-input weighted general ability of daily living index

ADLs	Weighting
Ability to eat by self	1.25
Ability to get to bed by self	0.90
Ability to get to toilet by self	1.37
Ability to wash by self	0.16
Ability to undress by self	0.09
Ability to shop by self	0.27
Ability to prepare meal by self	1.10
Ability to take medication by self	1.00
Ability to do household tasks by self	0.19

This index is the sum of the weighted number of problems users experience undertaking the activities of daily living listed above. The weights represent the relative influence of each of the tasks on total package costs, and were derived by multiple regression analysis.

This non-integer variable *WGADLSUM* has a range of 0.0 to 6.33 inclusive and is grouped into four bands of ADL ability levels to arrive at the final variable called WGADL_1 which is used in the analyses. The number and order of the bands is chosen to mirror the other general indicators such as INSERM classification and Isaacs and Neville need interval level.

WGADL_1	Very low ability	0<*WGADLSUM*<1.5825
	Low ability	1.5825<*WGADLSUM*<3.165
	High ability	3.165<*WGADLSUM*<4.7475
	Very high ability	4.7475<*wgadlsum*<6.33

5 Users' need-related circumstances and the response of informal caregivers: a comparison for the English and French samples

1. Need-related circumstances

The tables contrast the situation in England prior to the community care reforms of 1993 with that in France prior to the proposed introduction of the new *allocation autonomie* in 1995/6.

Table 1. Isaacs and Neville disability levels: proportions of persons by sample area

		Independent	*Long*	*Short*	*Critical*	*Total*
Area 1	row %	6.5	22.6	45.2	25.8	100.0
	no.	4	14	28	16	62
La Manche	row %	1.1	2.2	24.2	72.5	100.0
	no.	1	2	22	66	91
Area 2	row %	13.2	26.4	32.1	28.3	100.0
	no.	7	14	17	15	53
Athis Mons	row %	8.1	11.3	25.8	54.8	100.0
	no.	5	7	16	34	62
Area 3	row %	13.8	24.1	33.3	28.7	100.0
	no.	12	21	29	25	87
St Omer	row %	4.5	11.4	29.5	54.5	100.0
	no.	2	5	13	24	44

Difference between each sample areas, applying an exact Kruskal-Wallis Chi-square test:

Between Area 1 and La Manche: 0.0000
Between Area 2 and Athis Mons: 0.0033
Between Area 3 and St Omer: 0.0015

The English sample (Table 1), based on cases from the three areas described in section 1.3 of Chapter 4, are generally in lower dependency categories than the cases in the French sample. Within the French sites, there are much higher proportions of dependent people in La Manche. This may be due to factors such as the very rural nature of the area, with more scope for elderly people to be helped within an extended family which has not suffered either the migration noticeable in suburban areas such as Athis Mons, or the industrial past of St Omer, in the former mining area of Northern France.

When disability is measured following the POW QI score (Table 2), the English Area 3 appears to have a more dependent population than its French equivalent. Across all three English sites there are no cases in the very high ability range. This perhaps indicates how different

Table 2. POW QI weighted general ADL score: proportions of persons by sample area

		V. high ability	*High ability*	*Low ability*	*V. low ability*	*Total*
Area 1	row %		55.6	41.3	3.2	100.0
	no.		35	26	2	63
La Manche	row %	16.5	36.3	17.6	29.7	100.0
	no.	15	33	16	27	91
Area 2	row %		54.5	38.2	7.3	100.0
	no.		30	21	4	55
Athis Mons	row %	46.8	22.6	9.7	21.0	100.0
	no.	29	14	6	13	62
Area 3	row %		60.0	21.5	18.5	100.0
	no.		78	28	24	130
St Omer	row %	48.9	28.9	11.1	11.1	100.0
	no.	22	13	5	5	45

Difference between each sample areas, applying an exact Kruskal-Wallis Chi-square test:
Between Area 1 and La Manche: 0.5534
Between Area 2 and Athis Mons: 0.0012
Between Area 3 and St Omer: 0.0000

Table 3. Ability to perform personal care tasks:[a] proportions of persons by sample area

		Yes	Total
Area 1	row %	100.0	100.0
	no.	63	63
La Manche	row %	57.1	100.0
	no.	52	91
Area 2	row %	100.0	100.0
	no.	55	55
Athis Mons	row %	75.8	100.0
	no.	47	62
Area 3	row %	87.7	100.0
	no.	114	130
St Omer	row %	80.0	100.0
	no.	36	45

Difference between each sample areas, applying an exact Pearson Chi-square test:
Between Area 1 and La Manche: 0.0000
Between Area 2 and Athis Mons: 0.0000
Between Area 3 and St Omer: 0.2209

a Personal care tasks include the following: getting up and putting to bed; dressing and undressing; washing; nursing; toileting; changing incontinence pads.

ADLs affect differently costs in England and France. This would affect weights and therefore the derivation of the weighting score.

Most if not all the English sample were able to perform personal care tasks (Table 3). For the ability to perform household tasks (Table 4), the English sample again showed some signs of higher levels of functional ability than the French sample. This is further evidence of a difference in the need level of the French and English samples.

Tables 5 and 6 show significant differences in the proportions of cases with urinary incontinence between the English and French areas, between St Omer and Area 3.

Table 4. Ability to perform household tasks: proportions of persons by sample area

		Yes	Total
Area 1	row %	47.6	100.0
	no.	30	63
La Manche	row %	19.1	100.0
	no.	17	89
Area 2	row %	45.5	100.0
	no.	25	55
Athis Mons	row %	27.4	100.0
	no.	17	62
Area 3	row %	40.8	100.0
	no.	53	130
St Omer	row %	37.8	100.0
	no.	17	45

Difference between sample areas, applying an exact Pearson Chi-square test:
Between Area 1 and La Manche: 0.0097
Between Area 2 and Athis Mons: 0.2557
Between Area 3 and St Omer: 0.1651

Age distribution (Table 7) within the two national samples further supports the contrast in dependency, with a consistently higher pattern of over 85 year-olds in the French sites. However, the English samples include lower proportions of under 65s, with 8.1 per cent of the French sample in this category, against only 2 per cent of the British sample. This difference could reflect the time lapse between the collection of the French and English samples[1] since French workers involved in the collection of their data, who were also field workers of some experience, suggested that over the same period they had witnessed increasing dependency among their home care recipients.

Table 8 shows two of the French areas (Athis Mons and St Omer) with significantly higher proportions of cases in the 'separated/divorced/widowed' category when compared with their English equivalents or the third French site. This fact is likely to reflect local

1 The English sample collection data preceded the French sample collection by around ten years.

Table 5. Presence of urinary incontinence at first assessment

		Yes	Total
La Manche	%	18.0	100.0
	no.	16	89
Athis Mons	%	22.6	100.0
	no.	14	62
St Omer	%	9.3	100.0
	no.	4	43
Area 1	%	22.6	100.0
	no.	14	62
Area 2	%	27.3	100.0
	no.	15	55
Area 3	%	24.6	100.0
	no.	32	130

Difference between each sample area, applying an exact Kruskal-Wallis test:
Between Area 1 and La Manche: 0.4870
Between Area 2 and Athis Mons: 0.5591
Between Area 3 and St Omer: 0.0162

Table 6. Age by sample French and English sites at first assessment

		<55	55-65	65-75	75-85	85-95	Total
Area 1	row %	.0	3.3	34.4	49.2	13.1	100.0
	no.	0	2	21	30	8	61
La Manche	row %	1.1	3.3	24.4	44.4	26.7	100.0
	no.	1	3	22	40	24	90
Area 2	row %	.0	.0	23.6	52.7	23.6	100.0
	no.	0	0	13	29	13	55
Athis Mons	row %	4.8	9.7	11.3	33.9	40.3	100.0
	no.	3	6	7	21	25	62
Area 3	row %	1.1	1.1	28.7	59.8	9.2	100.0
	no.	1	1	25	52	8	87
St Omer	row %	2.2	4.4	28.9	44.4	20.0	100.0
	no.	1	2	13	20	9	45

Difference between each sample areas, applying a Kruskal-Wallis test:
Between Area 1 and La Manche: 0.0013
Between Area 2 and Athis Mons: 0.003
Between Area 3 and St Omer: 0.0007

Table 7. Marital status: proportions of persons by matched area

		Single	*Married*	*Separated/ divorced/ widowed*	*Total*
Area 1	row %	9.5	41.3	49.2	100.0
	no.	6	26	31	63
La Manche	row %	8.8	42.9	48.4	100.0
	no.	8	39	44	91
Area 2	row %	5.5	36.4	58.2	100.0
	no.	3	20	32	55
Athis Mons	row %	3.3	21.3	75.4	100.0
	no.	2	13	46	61
Area 3	row %	1.5	65.4	33.1	100.0
	no.	2	85	43	130
St Omer	row %	4.5	25.0	70.5	100.0
	no.	2	11	31	44

Difference between each sample areas, applying a Chi-squared test:
Between Area 1 and La Manche: 0.9754
Between Area 2 and Athis Mons: 0.0085
Between Area 3 and St Omer: 0.0000

socio-economic factors, such as the increased mortality of retired miners in St Omer, or the migratory suburban population in Athis Mons.

The national comparison for housing characteristics and tenure shows some significant differences between each of the pairs of matched areas. In general, English areas show better housing standards, with significantly higher proportions of centrally heated accommodation and inside toilets. Conversely, significantly higher proportions of French users stated that they were living in their own home.

2. Informal care and needs

What and how much help is provided by informal carers is of particular relevance to the French sample because of the presence of the *obligation alimentaire.* It will be remembered that it requires ascendant and

Table 8. Presence of central heating (main source): proportions of persons by matched area

		Central heating	Total
Area 1	row %	61.9	100.0
	no.	39	63
La Manche	row %	50.6	100.0
	no.	43	85
Area 2	row %	49.1	100.0
	no.	27	55
Athis Mons	row %	41.0	100.0
	no.	25	61
Area 3	row %	63.2	100.0
	no.	55	87
St Omer	row %	65.0	100.0
	no.	26	40

Difference between each sample areas, applying a Chi-squared test:
Between Area 1 and La Manche: 0.0526
Between Area 2 and Athis Mons: 0.1015
Between Area 3 and St Omer: 0.1550

descendant members of the family to care for their dependent elderly relative, or to pay for their institutional care should that be used. This widely-drawn legal obligation contrasts with the situation in Great Britain, where there is only a legal maintenance requirement between spouses or parents for their children while the latter are not yet of the legal age of responsibility. This requirement under the terms of *obligation alimentaire* can impose a severe strain on adult children. Indeed, these would be expected to contribute to the cost if their parents were to enter institutional care but lacked the financial resources and hence would otherwise be dependent on *aide sociale*. The provision of *aide sociale* for domiciliary care, however, is not affected by a requirement under *obligation alimentaire*. One would hypothesise that the two measures combined should have a powerful incentive effect on families to prevent their parents from entering institutional care. Equally, though, it could prevent a unified approach to the integration of funding of institutional and domiciliary care provision, since the higher real

Table 9. Client living in own home: proportions of persons by matched area

		Yes	Total
Area 1	row %	49.2	100.0
	no.	31	63
La Manche	row %	63.7	100.0
	no.	58	91
Area 2	row %	67.3	100.0
	no.	37	55
Athis Mons	row %	77.4	100.0
	no.	48	62
Area 3	row %	41.4	100.0
	no.	36	87
St Omer	row %	82.2	100.0
	no.	37	45

Difference between each sample areas, applying a Chi-squared test:
Between Area 1 and La Manche: 0.0267
Between Area 2 and Athis Mons: 0.0782
Between Area 3 and St Omer: 0.0000

Table 10. Accessibility of WC by French site at first assessment

		Inside, same level	*Inside, with steps*	*Outside, same level*	*Outside, no steps*	*Total*
La Manche	%	78.8	9.4	9.4	2.4	100.0
	no.	67	8	8	2	85
Athis Mons	%	90.2	8.2	.0	1.6	100.0
	no.	55	5	0	1	61
St Omer	%	78.6	.0	16.7	4.8	100.0
	no.	33	0	7	2	42
Total	%	82.4	6.9	8.0	2.7	100.0
	no.	155	13	15	5	188

Difference between all areas, applying a Chi-squared test: p=0.0000

Table 11. Presence of inside WC by English site

		Yes	Total
Area 1	%	98.4	100.0
	no.	62	63
Area 2	%	96.4	100.0
	no.	53	55
Area 3	%	96.6	100.0
	no.	84	87
Total	%	97.1	100.0
	no.	199	205

Difference between all areas, applying an exact Chi-squared test: p=0.1036

Difference between each sample, applying an exact Chi-squared test (inside toilet versus outside toilet):
Between La Manche and Area 1: 0.0171
Between Athis Mons and Area 2: 0.4609
Between St Omer and Area 3: 0.0001

cost of shelter-with-care is masked by the contributions made under *obligation alimentaire*. Thus, despite a policy of favouring home care, residential care may appear cheaper to the *aide sociale* budget than the provision of enhanced domiciliary care when considered in isolation. The fact remains, though, that there is no conclusive evidence of the effects of *obligation alimentaire* on the rate of entry into institutional care, so that its influence remains uncertain.

In view of the potential importance of the *obligation alimentaire*, the tables for both national samples are defined on the basis of the relationship of the informal helper within the *obligation alimentaire*. Those who would be liable to be included within its definition, in either the English or French sample, are defined as 'close relatives'; those outside the terms of *obligation alimentaire* are covered by the term 'other relative' (Tables 12 and 13 respectively).

Perhaps not surprisingly, in two of the three French samples, La Manche and Athis Mons, there was a high input from close relatives (Table 12). This was not true, however, of the third French site, St Omer. The explanation might lie in the immigration into the area of coalmine workers in earlier times, linked to the health problems associated with that industry, with a high mortality rate among its retired workers. Further support for this can be seen in the marital status table (Table

Table 12. Help from close relative: proportions of persons by sample area

		Yes	Total
Area 1	row %	27.0	100.0
	no.	17	63
La Manche	row %	53.8	100.0
	no.	49	91
Area 2	row %	36.4	100.0
	no.	20	55
Athis Mons	row %	53.2	100.0
	no.	33	62
Area 3	row %	23.8	100.0
	no.	31	130
St Omer	row %	11.1	100.0
	no.	5	45

Difference between each sample area, applying an exact Pearson Chi-square test:
Between Area 1 and La Manche: 0.0015
Between Area 2 and Athis Mons: 0.0938
Between Area 3 and St Omer: 0.0869

8) in the previous section. The proportion of widowed or divorced users in St Omer (70.5 per cent) is comparable to that in Athis Mons (75.4 per cent), but Athis Mons has more close relatives providing informal care inputs (53.2 per cent compared with 11.1 per cent for St Omer). Generally, Table 13 shows a very low involvement in the caring role from other relatives in both national samples, with other relatives in La Manche providing the higher proportion of informal care (11.0 per cent).

Table 14, which shows the presence of help from outside the family, is interesting because much is often made in France of the Anglo-Saxon enthusiasm for volunteer helpers. However, the evidence of this study is that the input in France from non-relatives is higher. This might be exaggerated since this category includes non-relatives being paid as helpers but not formally employed by an agency. Alternatively, the explanation might lie in the effects of the notable use of fiscal and cash allowances in the French system, which could serve to mobilise this category of helper.

Table 13. Help from other relative: proportions of persons by sample area

		Yes	Total
Area 1	row %	4.8	100.0
	no.	3	63
La Manche	row %	11.0	100.0
	no.	10	91
Area 2	row %		100.0
	no.		55
Athis Mons	row %	8.1	100.0
	no.	5	62
Area 3	row %	3.1	100.0
	no.	4	130
St Omer	row %		100.0
	no.		45
Total	%	2.3	100.0
	no.	4	175

Difference between each sample area, applying an exact Pearson Chi-square test:
Between Area 1 and La Manche: 0.2414
Between Area 2 and Athis Mons: 0.2117
Between Area 3 and St Omer: 0.2017

Table 15 compares the presence of informal help in the French and English samples by levels of dependency. There are no differences between the English and French samples in the proportions of low disability cases (long and medium interval levels) getting help from informal sources. However, higher proportions of the French cases in the short and critical interval levels get help from some informal source (44.1 per cent to 40.5 per cent for short interval, and 58.9 per cent to 41.1 per cent for critical interval need cases). This may reflect a higher concentration in France of informal help on those felt most likely to be otherwise at risk of entering institutional care and hence to impose an *obligation alimentaire* on their families. Although this would lend weight to the proposition that the presence of *obligation alimentaire* may be effective in mobilising informal help, its overall effect on the rate of institutionalisation remains unclear. Equally, the use of the cash allowance ACTP to mobilise non-formal help might be a factor. This issue is further explored in Chapter 6.

Table 14. Help from non-relative: proportions of persons by sample area

		Yes	*Total*
Area 1	row %	4.8	100.0
	no.	3	63
La Manche	row %	15.4	100.0
	no.	14	91
Area 2	row %		100.0
	no.		55
Athis Mons	row %	14.5	100.0
	no.	9	62
Area 3	row %	3.1	100.0
	no.	4	130
St Omer	row %	22.2	100.0
	no.	10	45

Difference between each sample area, applying an exact Pearson Chi-square test:
Between Area 1 and La Manche: 0.0644
Between Area 2 and Athis Mons: 0.0032
Between Area 3 and St Omer: 0.0002

Table 15. Presence of informal help with any tasks by Isaacs and Neville dependency level (English and French samples compared)

	Isaacs and Neville dependency level				
Presence of informal help	*Long interval*	*Medium interval*	*Short interval*	*Critical interval*	*Totals*
French sample:					
Numbers	3	4	22	73	102
Percentage	37.5	28.6	44.1	58.9	51.8
Total and overall percentage	8 (4.1)	14 (7.1)	51 (25.9)	124 (62.9)	197
English sample:					
Numbers	9	16	30	23	78
Percentage	39.1	32.7	40.5	41.1	38.6
Total and overall percentage	23(11.4)	49 (24.3)	74 (36.6)	56 (27.7)	202

Difference between samples, applying an exact Kruskal-Wallis test: p=0.0000

6 Formal agency response to needs and informal care

The first part of this chapter presents tables analysing the proportions of persons receiving formal help with various tasks in the matched areas for each country. The second part investigates the relationship and potential substitution between informal and formal sources in the provision of care.

1. Comparison of matched areas

Tables 16 and 17, which describe proportions receiving formal help for any task when the cases first applied for publicly-funded service, show much higher proportions of the French sample to have received formal services. This could be due to a speedier response in France. Certainly, there were integrated health and social care teams capable of fast response in two of the French sites. In those areas where services were integrated, 85.5 per cent and 93.3 per cent of cases were already receiving

Table 16. Presence of formal help with any tasks by Isaacs and Neville dependency level (English and French samples compared)

Presence of formal help	*Isaacs and Neville dependency level*				*Totals*
	Long interval	*Medium interval*	*Short interval*	*Critical interval*	
French sample:					
Numbers	4	11	38	92	145
Percentage	50.0	78.6	74.5	74.2	73.6
Total and overall percentage	8 (4.1)	14 (7.1)	51 (25.9)	124 (62.9)	197
English sample:					
Numbers	9	20	31	25	85
Percentage	39.1	40.8	41.9	44.6	42.1
Total and overall percentage	23 (11.4)	49 (24.3)	74 (36.6)	56 (27.7)	202

Table 17. Presence of formal help with any tasks: proportions of persons by area

		Yes	Total
Area 1	%	36.5	
	no.	23	63
La Manche	%	56.0	
	no.	51	91
Area 2	%	38.2	
	no.	21	55
Athis Mons	%	85.5	
	no.	53	62
Area 3	%	31.5	
	no.	41	130
St Omer	%	93.3	
	no.	42	45

Difference between sample areas, applying a Chi-squared test:
Between Area 1 and La Manche: 0.0077
Between Area 2 and Athis Mons: 0.0000
Between Area 3 and St Omer: 0.0000

services. In part, the typically fast response was to the higher dependency cases. This is more evident in the table for formal help with personal care than in the table for household tasks (Tables 18 and 19 respectively). La Manche had a lower proportion of users receiving help for household tasks than the English Area 1. Only for domiciliary meals and shopping (Tables 20 and 21 respectively) did the English sample show a consistently higher proportion of users receiving help by the time of first assessment. That may reflect the pattern of caseload dependency and marital status noted earlier.

Table 22 shows that more than 75 per cent of the recipients of ACTP had a member of the family other than their spouse providing care inputs. The result is of importance for predicting the effect of the new *prestation spécifique dépendance*. It suggests that the new benefit will be employed by those with extended families as a means to procure help from them, rather than to employ help from outside the family. The reverse is true for the English sample. None of the cases receiving attendance allowance (AA) had a relative other than a spouse caring. However, it was not possible to provide exactly comparable data for

Table 18. Presence of formal help with personal care: proportions of persons by area

		Yes	Total
Area 1	%	34.9	
	no.	22	63
La Manche	%	42.9	
	no.	39	91
Area 2	%	38.2	
	no.	21	55
Athis Mons	%	58.1	
	no.	36	62
Area 3	%	30.8	
	no.	40	130
St Omer	%	57.8	
	no.	26	45

Difference between sample areas, applying a Chi-squared test:
Between Area 1 and La Manche: 0.0823
Between Area 2 and Athis Mons: 0.0150

Table 19. Presence of formal help with housework: proportions of persons by area

		Yes	Total
Area 1	%	36.5	
	no.	23	63
La Manche	%	19.8	
	no.	18	91
Area 2	%	38.2	
	no.	21	55
Athis Mons	%	50.0	
	no.	31	62
Area 3	%	31.5	
	no.	41	130
St Omer	%	51.1	
	no.	23	45

Difference between sample areas, applying a Chi-squared test:
Between Area 1 and La Manche: 0.0107
Between Area 2 and Athis Mons: 0.0656

Table 20. Presence of formal help with meals: proportions of persons by area

		Yes	*Total*
Area 1	%	36.5	
	no.	23	63
La Manche	%	23.1	
	no.	21	91
Area 2	%	38.2	
	no.	21	55
Athis Mons	%	24.2	
	no.	15	62
Area 3	%	31.5	
	no.	41	130
St Omer	%	11.1	
	no.	5	45

Difference between sample areas, applying a Chi-squared test:
Between Area 1 and La Manche: 0.0566
Between Area 2 and Athis Mons: 0.0425

Table 21. Presence of formal help with shopping: proportions of persons by area

		Yes	*Total*
Area 1	%	36.5	
	no.	23	63
La Manche	%	15.4	
	no.	14	91
Area 2	%	38.2	
	no.	21	55
Athis Mons	%	32.3	
	no.	20	62
Area 3	%	31.5	
	no.	41	130
St Omer	%	28.9	
	no.	13	45

Difference between sample areas, applying a Chi-squared test:
Between Area 1 and La Manche: 0.0018
Between Area 2 and Athis Mons: 0.11231

Table 22. Presence of ACTP or attendance allowance by presence of relative other than spouse

	Presence of ACTP (at second assessment)	*Presence of AA (at first assessment)*
Relative other than spouse as helper		
Percentage	46.5	0.0
Numbers	33	0
Total	71	34
No helper or helper is non-relative or spouse		
Percentage	17.8	12.8
Numbers	8	6
Total	45	47
Total numbers	116	81

the English cases, since the information was collected at the first round only, and was limited to consideration of the spouse as the only potential informal family helper.

2. Do services in kind displace informal care?

2.1. Displacement, cost escalation, and the community care reform

Fear of escalating costs due first to the 'substitution' of publicly-subsidised care for informal care has long been a major policy influence.

In England, the Elizabethan 'Old' Poor Law allocated the responsibility for care of elderly parents to their children. The household means test was its powerful expression in the inter-war years. However, the unpopularity of the household means test caused the legislation of 1948 to apply a much narrower set of tests, and encouraged the development of publicly-subsidised social services.

The development of the publicly-subsidised social services make it more likely that formal services will displace informal caregiving, whether by family or by neighbours, it is suggested. In the UK of the 1970s, the sociologist Philip Abrams argued: 'there is impressive evidence to confirm the existence, hitherto, of a negative relationship between care provided *by* the community for its own members, and care provided *in* the community by public authorities: that is, the latter erodes the former' (Abrams, 1977, p.136).

Abrams argued that the provision of informal care was less worthwhile for general members of the community and, by extension, kith and kin. Abrams' argument was based on that by Hirsch (1977), who argued that the increasing value of time, and the uncertainty of reciprocity in a geographically mobile society, make individual investment in caring with the expectation of reciprocity later, appear increasingly risky. The cost to the individual of established services seems less. The argument was elaborated in Qureshi et al. (1989). The rise in the real value of earnings had increased the opportunity cost of time. Therefore, there was a growing incentive to substitute other sources of satisfaction for those requiring for their production much time in relation to other inputs. Looking after an elderly relative can often be an extremely time-consuming means of producing psychological satisfaction (or reducing dissatisfaction). Moreover, the productivity of informal care activities in terms of psychological benefits has probably not increased as much as the productivity in many other activities, despite the invention of the telephone, the vacuum cleaner, and the washing machine. Owen had found that for the US during the first six decades of the century, productivity in much non-work activity increased at much the same rate as in work activity, and that these non-work activities tended to be preferred by persons of higher income. Therefore, Qureshi et al. argued, the productivity of informal caring may have increased less than that of other non-work activity. So the psychological benefit from looking after an elderly relative had become more expensive in relation to the benefits from other non-work, and so one might expect a substitution of these other activities for caring.

There were other arguments. Hirsch (1977) postulated a 'commercialisation effect', whereby only what could be produced in marketable packages would be supplied. Titmuss (1968) argued that there was a link between the kind of motivation and the quality of what was produced. He argued that, once started, commercialisation would be irresistible. Paraphrasing the Titmuss argument, Leach (1971) referred to Gresham's Law: 'It is as true of moral values as it is of economics, that bad money drives out good.' However, as Arrow (1972) asserted,

Titmuss did not give a convincing reason why commercialisation would be irresistible.

The UK was only one country in which there was the fear of displacement. The same was true in the United States. Brody and Brody (1985) linked the fear to what they called a myth that families do not take care of the elderly. For 30 years, research has proved otherwise. The UK was not alone in the fear and its policy expression. No doubt, it is one reason why countries governed by the Napoleonic code retain an *obligation alimentaire* to this day.

Restricting provision to less attractive institutional care was a means used to curb demand. Chadwick's New Poor Law defined the principle of 'less eligibility', and imposed the 'workhouse test' as a means of securing it. Indeed, the provision of care mainly in institutions — entailing the loss of autonomy itself, the psychologically repugnant acceptance of entry as a rite of irreversible passage to dependency and death — rather than the provision of much more attractive care in the home, has always been linked with checking the escalation of public costs. We have seen how demand for the new more attractive home care services grew during the first year of the full operation of the reformed community care, with serious consequences for the relationship of finance and demand during the second year in some areas. Although the regimes of standard forms of residential and nursing homes have almost entirely precluded the input of care from family and others who would be major sources of care effort were the disabled person a recipient of home care, availability of publicly-funded support at a high level only in institutions had undoubtedly restrained demand in the past.

The near-universality of policy trends during the last decade suggests that major reform of the community care systems is almost inevitable. Evers talks about its features in many European countries in their treatment of 'the issue of welfare mix'. The point, they argue, is not that welfare is increasingly being produced in different sectors. It is that the features of each of the sectors have changed, and that 'new citizen rights' and 'micro-solidarities' have developed. These call into question the traditional design of policies and services:

> they should no longer see themselves as state-centred policies, but policies and processes which aim at a better interaction of a plurality of different actors and sectors ... differences and con-

> troversies are less and less about whether one of the sectors is of importance or should play a role, but rather about the characteristics of its contributions and *how to tie it in* (our italics) (Evers, 1994, pp.17-18).

Two of the four challenges which they identify are: 'from standardised formal welfare services to negotiated forms of community-based care, mixing formal and informal elements' (p.21), and 'from tacit use to planned involvement of women's informal care' (p.23). Policy reforms seek to make the formal support systems work around the needs and wishes of users and their networks, and to offer a choice of staying in their own homes to persons who would otherwise have been forced either to enter residential modes of care or be offered only inadequate support in the home. These aims are not just the highest common factors of the goals of care policy. They are also its most revolutionary feature, when viewed in the historical context of the relationships between the workhouse test and the prevention of cost escalation.

Commentators have spoken of the sensitivity to the potential 'substitution' of formal for informal care among politicians and other policy-makers. Reformers have battled against the 'substitution' argument in post-war academe. Linsk et al. (1992) describe how the fear of it was present among officials in American states in their appreciations of payments for family care.

Much gerontological analysis has been a direct response to these fears. In this country, it was the group which produced the founding works of British gerontology and classics of family sociology post-war (Shanas et al., 1968; Shanas 1979; Young and Willmott, 1957; Townsend, 1962) — the Institute of Community Studies at Bethnal Green — who first argued that families were not abandoning their elderly members, but were adapting their care inputs to changes in circumstances. The theme, oft-repeated here, was taken up in the United States with, among other studies, the cross-national investigation of the late 1960s, and has been maintained as a *Leitmotif* of argument ever since. Every generation redefines the issue in terms of the economic and social changes of the time, contemporary writers doing so in terms of marital disruption and divorce, greater participation of women in paid employment, the smaller size and increasing geographic mobility of families, and changing expectations of women.

Thus, in outline, do 'substitution', escalation of costs to public funds, and a reform of community care which takes into account the rights of citizens to live at home, interrelate.

2.2. *Displacement, 'substitution', and related concepts*

The word 'substitution' is commonly used in the Anglo-Saxon literature to describe the displacement of inputs from informal carers by inputs from agencies. One reason why the evidence about displacement is so unsatisfactory is that the word 'substitution' is used vaguely, and to describe different phenomena.

One general meaning is the reduction of care inputs by informal caregivers which occurs because formal agencies provide the services which the informal carers would otherwise undertake. There is the replacement of informal inputs whose confirmed contribution was at the beginning of the period expected of caregivers of that degree of relational propinquity and other circumstances. The second meaning is the assumption of care roles by formal agencies in the absence, or subsequent to the loss, of others in the informal social network from whom the inputs would be expected. So the first meaning implied that there would be equivalent care from the informal sector in the absence of the formal inputs. The second meaning implies that the person would not receive care from that source. The data collected for the project allow analysis only of the first.

Substitution can take two basic forms: (i) within a mode of care and (ii) between modes of care. Most studies investigate only the former: for instance, substitution of inputs into household tasks by agencies for inputs into the same tasks by relatives for elderly persons who continue to live in their own home. The second is the replacement of a mode of care which draws extensively on informal sources for inputs by one which draws mainly on formal sources. An example is the substitution of care in a residential facility for care at home.

Within-mode substitution

The context of within-mode substitution is the hierarchy-compensatory argument. One form is the replacement by formal service inputs of informal inputs which at the beginning of the period over which the process is studied are not expected of carers of that gender, degree of relational propinquity, set of other social obligations, or history of family relationships. That is, the shift in source of care inputs are consonant with equity criteria as defined at the beginning of the period, and before the definition of the equity criteria themselves are contaminated by changes due to change in practice itself. The equity criteria should take into account the hierarchy-compensatory argument: the displacement to persons with more distant relationships of tasks for which the expectation would be performance by someone nearer in the absence of the nearer relations.

The argument has been well developed in the new world (Shanas, 1968; Cantor, 1980). Its existence has been argued in the British literature (Qureshi and Walker, 1989; Qureshi, 1990). It has been postulated also in France, where Curtis et al. concluded:

> the pattern of instrumental [ADL/IADL-related] support reported in this paper for three French regions seems to have similar broad characteristics to the patterns observed in other countries. Most notably, the evidence from this study corresponds with other findings which demonstrate a hierarchical structure of care givers in which the dominant source of help is from members of the family (1992, p.346).

Between-mode substitution

Jette et al. (1995) postulate the three patterns in a study of entry to residential facilities for long-term care. Table 23 extends the same idea to our distinction between within-mode and between-mode substitution.

The 'main effect' distinguished in the table would be substitution in either of two types of model. One type would be the models in which the utilisation of the institutions were treated as an inverse indicator of outputs: perhaps days of adequate care living at home, analogous to active life years in the measurement of health outcomes. The other type would be models in which home and informal care (individually or collectively) substitute for inputs in residential modes of care in the production of unspecified dimensions of welfare which are causally further along the production process than modes of care. The 'buffering effect' could be considered to be a substitution in a model which treated

Table 23. Three patterns of within-mode and between-mode substitution[a]

'Main effect' pattern

Within-mode substitution:

Inputs of formal in-home services replace informal inputs in the improvement of quality of life and care.

Between-mode substitution:

Inputs of formal care in cases in which inputs of informal care at home reduce the probability that a mode of care is replaced by a mode which has smaller inputs of informal care; for instance, home care with inputs from relatives is replaced by entry to institutions with less input from relatives. The inputs of formal or informal care directly and independently reduce the probability of entry.

'Buffering' pattern

Within-mode substitution:

Helping persons to cope at home, the inputs of formal care buffer the effects of disability, cognitive impairment, specific health conditions and other risk factors, so increasing the productivities of informal care inputs on aspects of the quality of life and care of the person supported. The inputs of formal care moderate the effects of the risk factors.

Between-mode substitution:

Helping the persons to cope at home, the inputs of informal *or* formal care buffer the effects of risk factors on the probability of entry into institutions (Wan and Weissert, 1981). The effect of the risk factors is reduced more, the greater are the inputs of informal or formal care.

'Supplementation' pattern

Within-mode substition:

Inputs of formal in-home services replace informal inputs.

Between-mode substitution:

Inputs of formal care increase the effectiveness of informal care in reducing the probability of entry to institutions by relieving strain on carers (perhaps by allowing caregivers to undertake less onerous tasks, perhaps by reducing their total input), so that the receipt of formal services in addition to informal care reduces the probability of entry.

a The study of within-mode and between-mode substitutions is complicated when one takes into account cash subsidies by the informal sector as well as services in kind. Informal care hours might be reduced, but the informal sector might be paying for the increase in the hours of services. Similarly, the hours of informal inputs might be reduced by an admission to residential modes of care, but the informal carers might have increased their subsidy to the dependent person.

the risk factors as inverse inputs,[1] since the effect of the care inputs would be to affect the impact of these risk factors. The 'supplementation effect' could be considered a substitution effect either in a model in which days of adequate care at home rather than residential care were the output, or in which community and residential care inputs were inputs in the production of outcomes further along the process of producing welfare of value in its own right.

It is too easy for policy-makers to interpret anecdotal evidence about the second definition as if it were evidence about the first. That can only feed populist fears about the price that it is necessary to pay for improvements in the wellbeing of welfare beneficiaries. The effect can be to create a smokescreen of political sentiment which makes it difficult to create clear new equity principles so as to redefine rights and obligations in the light of new values and contingencies.

The data collected allow only the investigation of within-mode substitution. The mode on which the analysis is focused is community-based service.

Also the evidence is indirect and exclusively about inputs. The argument makes clear that the direct estimation of substitution requires that informal care is displaced by formal care, allowing for changes in outcomes that would require evidence also about outcomes. The basis for the estimation of substitution should in principle be models showing the relations between inputs and outcomes. The data available do not allow their estimation.

---

1 They are handled thus in some production function models of human services, as in the production of welfare approach (Davies and Challis, 1981, 1986; Davies and Knapp, 1981; Knapp, 1984). They are there called 'quasi-inputs'. However, there the full power of the production of welfare model cannot be exploited unless there are ratio scale measures of inputs and at least interval scale measures of outputs. Secondly, production of welfare models aim to cover all the important interrelated inputs and outputs. Thirdly, it is usually the case that the models are interested in substitution in both directions: the partial replacement of informal for formal care (as might happen in some cases when formal services are removed or reduced in quantity at times of budget crisis) as well as that of formal for informal care (as is postulated by Jette et al., 1995).

Box 8. *Definitions of substitution-related indicators*

i) Absolute measure

Definition 1: whether substitution

Has there been a reduction in the amount of informal help? If yes, has there been an increase in the amount of formal help hours? If yes to both questions, then substitution took place. Let F1 and I1 be formal and informal hours at time one respectively. Let F2 and I2 be their equivalent at time 2. Let ΔF and ΔI be the changes between time 1 and time 2. There is substitution if:

$$\Delta F>0 \text{ and } \Delta I<0.$$

ii) Relative measures

Let H1 be the total amount of hours of help in time 1 (H1 = T1 + I1). Let $\delta F=\Delta F/H1$, and $\delta I=\Delta I/1$.

Definition 2: for the cases for which substitution has taken place, what is the overall change in amount of help relative to the initial overall amount of help?

$$|\delta I|+\delta F$$

Definition 3: for cases for which substitution has taken place, what is the size of the change in informal help relative to the change in formal help?

$$|\delta I|/\delta F$$

2.3. *Displacement-related indicators*

Box 8 defines indicators. They consist of indicators of whether a replacement of formal for informal care has occurred, and indicators of how great was the displacement.

The approach follows the work of Tennstedt et al. (1993). It defines substitution as occurring when an increase in formal service between data collection rounds is accompanied by a decrease in informal care hours. However, that definition does not indicate *how much* substitution takes place for those cases for whom there was substitution: on average, how many hours of informal care are diminished. Likewise, it does not indicate what proportion of the increase in formal care hours is accounted for by reductions in informal care hours. Again, the definition in itself neither takes into account changes in the need-related circumstances of the person with the handicap, nor the situation of the social support network which is the source of the informal helping input. The indicators and their analysis reported here cover both criticisms.

Table 24. Whether substitution takes place (yes if $\Delta F>0$ and $\Delta I<0$)

Definition 1 *Presence of substitution*	*1st and 2nd assessment*	*Period between:* *2nd and 3rd assessment*	*Overall*
All tasks			
Number	7	11	18
Per cent	8.4	17.7	12.4
Total	83	62	145
Personal care tasks			
Number	8	7	15
Per cent	9.6	11.3	10.3
Total	83	62	145
Housework tasks			
Number	1	4	5
Per cent	1.2	6.5	3.4
Number	83	62	145
Help with meals			
Number	3	4	7
Per cent	3.6	6.5	4.8
Total numbers	83	62	145

Following Tennstedt et al. in another respect, they also allow for the norms which influence the probabilities with which different forms of help is sought from persons, as these have been described for instance in the hierarchy of obligations among informal carers developed by Qureshi and Walker (1989; Qureshi, 1990), or the arguments about the specialisation of persons with different relationships, and between formal and informal care, in the nature and content of what they provide, and how they provide it. An honourable exception is Tennstedt et al. (1993, pp.607-8), who take into account 'specialisation within informal care': the substitution of formal services for informal care in one area of assistance accompanied by an increase of informal hours in one or more other areas of assistance. Our analysis allows for displacement of

Table 25. Relative measures of substitution for all cases and all tasks

Values	Def.2: |δ|+δF Freq.	%	Def.3: |δ|/δF Values	Freq.	%
0.00	127	88.10	0.00	127	88.10
0.00	1	.69	0.02	1	.69
0.02	1	.69	0.04	1	.69
0.05	1	.69	0.20	1	.69
0.08	1	.69	0.22	1	.69
0.10	1	.69	0.23	1	.69
0.11	1	.69	0.61	1	.69
0.13	1	.69	0.75	1	.69
0.22	1	.69	0.79	1	.69
0.26	1	.69	1.00	1	.69
0.29	1	.69	1.20	1	.69
0.36	1	.69	6.98	1	.69
0.84	1	.69	7.74	1	.69
1.01	1	.69	8.04	1	.69
1.05	1	.69	9.90	1	.69
1.20	1	.69	10.50	1	.69
1.37	1	.69	11.11	1	.69
1.67	1	.69	12.96	1	.69
3.74	1	.69	14.91	1	.69
Total numbers	145	100		145	145

activity between personal care, household tasks, and other care activities.

2.4. *Results*

The evidence for France is compatible with only a low degree of displacement of formal for informal care input. This is the case for all three definitions of substitution, for all particular tasks, and for all assessments.

Table 24 reports the results for Definition 1. It suggests that the proportions of cases which show substitution always remain below 18.0 per cent whatever the task or period. The highest proportions are for

Table 26. Relative measures of substitution only for cases with no changes in disability (all tasks)

	Def.2: $\lvert\delta\rvert + \delta F$		*Def.3: $\lvert\delta\rvert / \delta F$*		
Values	*Freq.*	*%*	*Values*	*Freq.*	*%*
0.00	59	88.10	0.00	59	88.10
0.00	1	1.50	0.20	1	1.50
0.05	1	1.50	0.61	1	1.50
0.10	1	1.50	0.75	1	1.50
0.11	1	1.50	1.00	1	1.50
0.22	1	1.50	6.98	1	1.50
0.26	1	1.50	7.74	1	1.50
0.36	1	1.50	9.90	1	1.50
1.05	1	1.50	14.91	1	1.50
Total	67	100		67	100

all tasks and personal care tasks: 12.4 per cent and 10.3 per cent of the cases respectively overall. However, the substitution effect seems to increase between the second and third assessments (from 8.4 per cent between the first and second assessment to 17.7 per cent between the second and third assessments for all tasks). Perhaps formal and informal helpers take time to adjust to changes in each other's level of help.

Table 25 presents the frequency distributions for the relative measures including all tasks and for all cases, including those whose level of ability to perform daily living tasks had changed over the period. A value of unity by Definition 2 means that the sum of the decrease in informal inputs plus the increase in formal inputs (the overall amount of change in hours of help) is equivalent to the initial amount of help the case was getting. A value greater than one would then suggest an even greater volume of change due to the substitution effect. A value of unity for Definition 3 means that the volume of informal help has decreased by the same amount that levels of formal help increased. If this rate is greater than unity, then the informal help would have decreased by more than the formal help increased. The range suggests that there may have been extensive substitution for some cases. Indeed, for 7 out of the 18 cases presenting traces of substitution, the rate of overall volume of change is close to unity (def.2>.8). Moreover, for 10 cases the decrease in informal help surpasses the increase in formal

Figure 2. Model of relations between (1) initial need-related circumstances; (2) initial help from informal caregivers; (3) allocations of formal services; (4) changes in need-related circumstances; (5) changes in informal help; (6) changes in formal services; (7) 'outcomes'

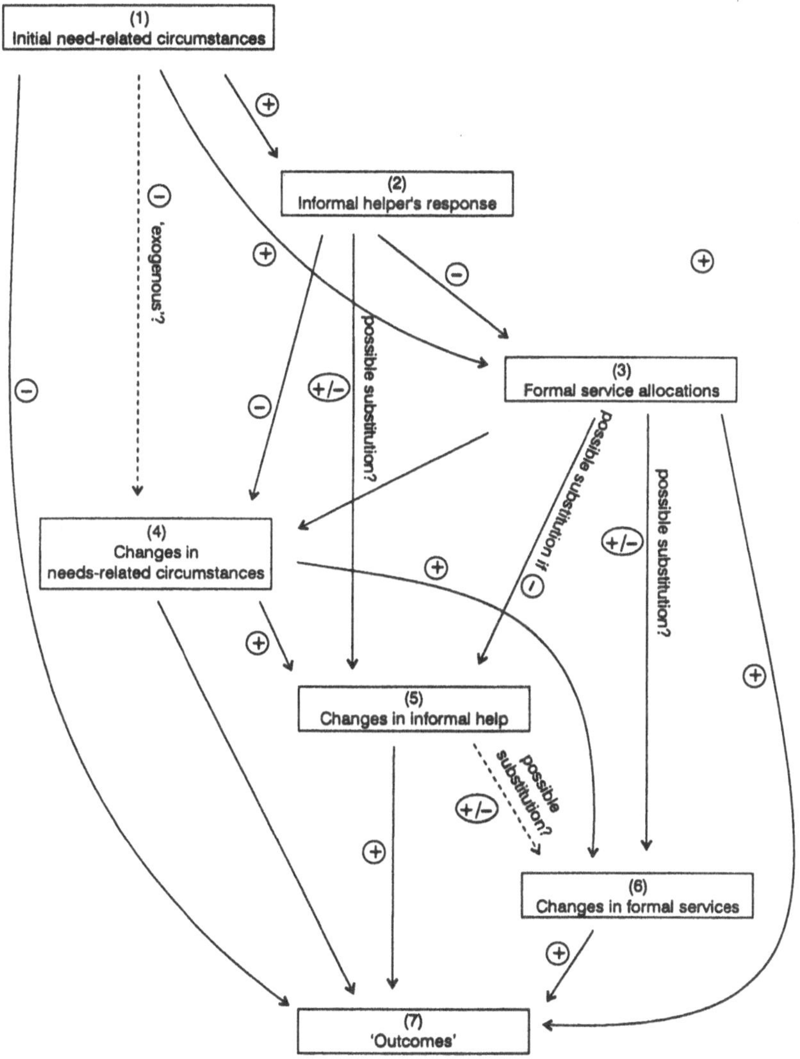

Principal outcomes are: (i) substitution of formal for informal care, (ii) admission/placement in institutions etc., and (iii) death.

help (def.3>1). This means that for such cases the total amount of help (both informal and formal) has decreased, even after the increase in formal inputs. Nevertheless, the evidence in Table 25 may exaggerate the prevalence of substitution.

Table 26 reports frequency distributions for the relative measures for all tasks, and among the cases with no changes in disability.[2] Here again the evidence of substitution effect remains very limited: only for 6.0 per cent of the population did the overall change in the amount of help relative to the initial overall amount (def.2) exceed 20 per cent. Also, only for 7.5 per cent of the population did the decrease in informal help exceed the increase in levels of formal help (def.3>1).

2.5. *Model form*

Another method was used to illuminate the degree of displacement: the statistical modelling of substitutions through time. Patterns of utilisation of care from formal and informal sources were related to need-related circumstances at the point of entry to the system and over the two subsequent six-month periods. (Numbers were too small to permit analysis for the third period.) The general form of the model is outlined in Figure 2. It will be seen that the form is recursive.

- It is assumed that the inputs of informal care are a response to need-related circumstances which, in turn, influence the level of formal care. However, the inputs of formal care are in part directly influenced by the need-related circumstances.
- The levels of informal and formal care are postulated to influence changes in needs, it being argued that informal and formal support inputs have a 'buffering' effect, reducing the impact of need-related circumstances on outcomes (Jette et al., 1995).

The distributions of inputs are characterised by a large number of observations with a value of zero, with considerable variance about

---

2 We reduce in this way the risk of interpreting as evidence of substitution changes in levels of help due to changes in levels of need. Nevertheless, many other factors other than changes in disability may account for some of the substitution, as for instance changes in the availability of informal helpers.

Table 27. Direction and significance of interactions between need-related circumstances and amount of informal and formal help through time (any tasks)

Explanatory variables	*Informal help t1 Sign (p)*	*Formal help t1 Sign (p)*	*Decrease disability Sign (p)*	*Increase inf. help Sign (p)*	*Increase form. help Sign (p)*
Housebound t1	+ .0032				
Disability level t1	+ .0151	+ .0000	+ .0198	+ .0132	+ .0048
Changes in disability (t2-t1)				+ .1297	+ .0021
User lives alone t1	- .0143	+ .0215			
Informal carer is close female relative	+ .0000				
User is male					+ .0287
La Manche		- .0002			
Hours informal help companionship t1					+ .0285
Hours informal help housework t1				- .0087	- .0309
Changes inf. help housework (t2-t1)					- .0244
Hours informal help personal care t1		- .0024	- .2310		- .0358
Hours formal help companionship t1			+ .0712		
Hours formal help personal care t1			- .0728		
Hours formal help housework t1				-.0587	

that level. Regression analysis requires distributions of the dependent variable approximating to normality. Therefore the analysis used logistic regression to predict whether or not there was an input at first assessment. It did so for three kind of tasks (housework, personal care and all tasks), and for whether there was an increase in the level of input between first and second assessments.

Table 28. Direction and significance of interactions between need-related circumstances and amounts of informal and formal help through time (personal care tasks)

Explanatory variables	*Informal help t1 Sign (p)*	*Formal help t1 Sign (p)*	*Decrease disability Sign (p)*	*Increase inf. help Sign (p)*	*Increase form. help Sign (p)*
Housebound t1	+ .0003				
Incontinence t1	+ .2038				
Disability level t1	+ .0309	+ .0000	+ .0198	+ .0068	
Changes in disability (t2-t1)				+ .0057	+ .0438
User lives alone t1	- .0016	+ .0321			
User is male				+ .1065	+ .0083
La Manche	+ .0002	- .0008		+ .0047	
Hours informal help personal care t1			- .2310	- .0072	
Hours informal help housework t1					- .0256
Hours formal help companionship t1			+ .0712		- .0237
Hours formal help personal care t1			- .0728		
Hours formal help housework t1					+ .0348
No. of meals formal help t1				- .0500	+ .0409

Need-related circumstances are postulated to have a positive effect on hours, so that the hypotheses have a single tail. Informal care is postulated to have a negative effect on the inputs of formal care.

2.6. *Model results*

Tables 27, 28 and 29 summarise the results of the modelling of the interactions between informal help, formal help and need-related circumstances for all tasks, personal care tasks and housework tasks respectively. The dependent variables are located at the top of the tables, and the explanatory variables to the left of the table. Within the table

Table 29. Direction and significance of interactions between need-related circumstances and amounts of informal and formal help through time (housework tasks)

Explanatory variables	*Informal help t1 Sign (p)*	*Formal help t1 Sign (p)*	*Decrease disability Sign (p)*	*Increase inf. help Sign (p)*	*Increase form. help Sign (p)*
Age t1		+ .0409			
Cancer t1	+ .1029				
Disability level t1			+ .0198		
User in med.-low disab. group t1					- .0174
Changes in disability (t2-t1)				+ .0926	+ .1447
User lives alone t1	- .0023	+ .0321			
No. in household		- .0343			
Inf. carer is close female relative t1	+ .0003				
La Manche	- .0023	- .0000			+ .0072
Hours informal help housework t1		- .0030			- .0369
Changes in informal help housework				- .0034	- .0199
Hours informal help personal care t1			- .2310		- .0195
Hours informal help meals t1				+ .0004	+ .0073
Hours formal help companionship t1			+ .0712		+ .0348
Hours formal help personal care t1		- .0728			
No. of meals formal help t1					+ .0118

is shown the direction and significance of the correlation between the explanatory and dependent variables of the models.

The analysis of the results is divided into three main categories: first, the analysis of how need-related circumstances affect both formal and informal help; second, how levels of informal help and formal help interact with each other, and what that tells us about the potential for substitution of formal help for informal help; and finally, given the fact that La Manche is characterised by the use of ACTP, its presence as significant explanatory variable provides hints about the effects of ACTP on levels of formal and informal help.

This progression will be applied in the analysis of the results for any tasks, personal care tasks, and housework tasks.

Effects of need-related circumstances on levels of informal and formal help

Need-related circumstances seem to affect levels of help as one would predict:

Any tasks (Table 27)

- A client who is housebound has more chance of receiving informal help.
- Disability levels increase the chance of receiving formal and/or informal help. High levels of disability at first assessment are also associated with high probabilities of increase in the levels of informal and formal help between first and second assessment.
- A client living alone has more chance of receiving formal help and less chance of informal help.
- The presence of a close female in the household increases the chance of receiving informal help.
- A male client has more chance of having an increase in levels of formal help.

Personal care tasks (Table 28)

- A client who is housebound has more chance of receiving informal help.
- Incontinence increases the probability of receiving some informal help.
- Disability levels increase the chance of receiving formal and/or informal help as well as the probability of an increase in levels of formal help.
- A client living alone has less chance of receiving informal help and more chance of receiving formal help.

Housework tasks (Table 29)

• Age is positively correlated with the probabilities of receiving some formal help.

• A client suffering from cancer has more chance of receiving informal help.

• Deterioration in ability levels increases the chance of receiving an increase in levels of formal help and informal help.

• A client living alone has less chance of receiving informal help.

• Numbers in household decrease the chance of getting some formal help.

• The presence of a close female in the household increases the chance of receiving informal help.

Interactions between informal and formal help

The conclusions of this subsection are drawn from the shaded areas in the tables. In such areas one can read the direction and significance of the correlation between formal and informal help. Negative signs in the 'Formal help time 1' and 'Increase in formal help' columns are to be interpreted as evidence that formal services tune their inputs with the existing levels of input from informal sources. Negative signs on the column 'Increase in formal help' denote how the chance of an increase in informal help diminishes as the amount of formal help increases. Therefore, the presence of significant negative signs in the shaded area of this column denotes great scope for substitution effect. The variation in the pattern of informal and formal help due to changes in other need-related circumstances (e.g. changes in disability or availability of informal sources of help) should have been controlled for within the model.

Any tasks (Table 27)

• There is clear evidence that inputs from formal sources accommodate to the level of informal inputs.

• The probability of an increase in formal inputs at second assessment is significantly negatively correlated with the presence of informal help with housework, personal care, and with increases in the level of informal help with housework.

• Furthermore, the results show scope for substitution between informal help with all tasks and housework formal inputs. The likelihood of an increase in levels of informal help is significantly negatively correlated with levels of formal help with housework.

Personal care tasks (Table 28)

- There is some evidence of substitution between informal help with personal care tasks and formal help with meals.
- Formal help with personal care is less likely to increase if the input levels of informal help with housework increase.

Housework tasks (Table 29)

- There is no evidence of substitution between informal help with housework and formal inputs.
- However, initial levels of formal help with housework are negatively correlated with the presence and levels of informal help with housework, and with the levels of input from informal help with personal care.

La Manche: significantly different

La Manche appears significantly negatively associated with the presence of formal help. Therefore, clients from La Manche seem to be less likely to have formal help. This might be due to the fact that this formal help is performed by informal helpers paid with the ACTP. Although La Manche does not appear significantly positively related to the presence of informal help, this could still be true if the hours of care provided by informal carers were higher in La Manche than by those in St Omer or Athis Mons. Alternatively, La Manche may not show higher probabilities of receipt of informal care due to its slow allocation of ACTP.

La Manche is negatively correlated with the presence of formal help with personal care tasks (Table 28). Here, however, ACTP is positively correlated with the presence of informal help, as well as with the increase in levels of informal help.

La Manche is negatively correlated to both presence of formal and informal help with housework tasks, but positively correlated with increases in levels of formal help with housework (Table 29).

2.7. Conclusions

This section first compared the formal agency inputs in the matched areas in the two countries, allowing for variations in the handicap-related circumstances of individuals and the care inputs from 'informal caregivers'. There were some interesting contrasts. For instance, in England and Wales, recipients of attendance allowance tended not to have inputs from their informal social network other than from their spouses. In France, the ACTP was received mainly by persons with extended families, and was used to procure help from them. The result for France begs the question whether the new *prestation spécifique dépendance* would be used primarily to pay informal and near-informal helpers rather than service providers. Viewed in this light, the *prestation spécifique dépendance* might prove to make a connection between the development of the *chèque service* and the recruitment of help from organisations like *associations mandataires*, and become another French manifestation of what may be a trend towards the 'deformalisation of social care'. This was a facet of the Kent Community Care Project, the British case management experiment of the seventies (Davies and Challis, 1986; Qureshi et al., 1989), though a facet which ran counter to the cultures of British social services department and local authorities as a whole. The payment of neighbours and other quasi-informal helpers later became a feature of British development during the 1980s (Leat, 1988). In the Kent Community Care Project and many of the authority care arrangements of the following decade, the payments were for the performance of tasks in a contract of greater or lesser explicitness. This is a feature which distinguishes between some of the more recent developments. On the one hand, the highly popular cash option in the German long-term care insurance system does not imply strong contracts. On the other hand, the American consumer-directed models being adapted to meet the circumstances of an elderly rather than younger disabled population and to which federal attention has increasingly turned since the failure of the Clinton Act created a policy vacuum in the support of frail elderly people, do so to a greater extent, though to an extent which differs between the models.[3] The same is so for British proposals for direct

3 In consumer-directed models, public funds are allocated to the consumers, who themselves recruit and manage care to a greater degree than in conven-

payments. The nature of the relationship between the helper, the user and the funder is important because it is key to some of the concerns about such models: cost escalation, the risk of abuse and the technical difficulty of assuring quality, the dangers of reducing horizontal target efficiency (Davies, 1992).

The second theme of the section has been the likely degree of displacement of informal care inputs by agency-provided services. The discussion of sections 2.1 and 2.2 illustrated the degree to which this has been a concern of Anglo-Saxon policy analysis. However, it also illustrates that the analysis of evidence about it has been crude. The concepts used — in particular, 'substitution' and 'diversion' — have been too loosely defined, or defined in ways which disregard the complex patterns of social structures and processes which research has shown to underlie the realities being investigated. The section advances the discussion by first refining concepts and tying them to types of activity for whom gerontological argument would suggest differences in patterns, and then estimating different kinds of substitution/diversion-related effects, setting the estimates in the context of a model investigating the interdependence of flows of help from different sources with one another and with need-related circumstances through time.

The results do not suggest that the provision of services greatly reduces the inputs of informal care. There could be substitution for relatively few cases, whatever the task, and whatever the period. The more refined the analysis, the less prevalent and powerful were the substitutions compatible with its results. This is so although the general models discussed in sections 2.5 and 2.6 would be compatible with substitutions.

The study of potential substitution remains in its infancy. One reason is the inappropriateness of the analyses and evidence so far used. 'Substitution' is a concept borrowed from economics. It should be viewed in the context of the production of various welfare outcomes for beneficiaries using care inputs from different sources. In this 'production of welfare' context, its nature and extent can only be measured in the context of models which relate inputs to outcomes of evaluative sig-

---

tional case management-led or service-led models. The consumer- directed models vary in the extent of case management support provided to the consumers.

nificance in their own right. That requires more evidence than it was possible to collect in this study. There have been no attempts to estimate substitutions using production functions relating inputs to outcomes which take into account the complexity of social structures and processes, and treat substitution as a process through time, though some work on the Kent Community Care Project and its replications suggest that production functions could usefully be considered in this way.

A second reason is that some of the main forms of substitution effects can take a long time to develop. Some of the trends discussed in sections 2.1 and 2.2 occur only over long periods; for instance, the reduction of the costs of purchasing agency inputs rather than providing informal care. It might take years for the full effects to be felt of providing high standard home care rather than imposing what the Victorian English called the 'workhouse test' of 'less eligibility' — enforced incarceration in a workhouse with loss of the rights of citizenship, dignity and autonomy as well as a squalid material standard of living — to work through to changed norms and expectations in families. To assess these substitution effects, it would be necessary to examine substitutions for successive cohorts in a design which allowed the separation of effects of more or less attractive home care services.

7 Entry into institutions

For some, admission to a residential facility for long-term care can provide a more attractive physical environment and material standard of living than the alternative. People vary in the degree to which they would prefer to take the risks of continuing to live in the community than to sacrifice autonomy and treasured aspects of their ways of life. However, the results of research in the UK and other countries suggest that most would prefer adequate care in their own homes to care in residential homes, nursing homes and long-stay hospitals as they currently are. Research shows that, for many, admission to such institutions for long-term care is *faute de mieux* (Warburton, 1994). It also shows that the proportion of the population surviving to the fourth age who at some stage will be admitted to an institution for long-term care is substantial, although the proportion resident there at any one point in time is low. One estimate is that someone surviving until the age of 65 in the USA has a 42 per cent probability of spending time in a nursing home prior to their death (Kemper et al., 1991). In almost all countries, it is clear that too high a proportion of recipients of care have been forced to receive it in conventional institutions for long-term care, not in private households in the community, or living arrangements which provide social and psychological environments more like that of life at home.

For that reason alone, it is unsurprising that, in most countries, one important rationale for the subsidisation of home care is to make unwanted entry to an institution necessary for fewer persons (OECD, 1994). That is as true of British community care policy during the eighties and nineties as it is in France, for which section 1 in Chapter 1 illustrated the importance of the goal in formal statements of the objectives of services.

Therefore, one of the principal evaluative criteria for assessing the performance of a country's package of community care policy devices — home care services and cash payments to procure care inputs — is in practice the degree to which they reduce the utilisation of institutions for long-term care. This section compares the success of British and

French systems by this criterion, also assessing the effects of the provision of agency services and cash benefits for the procurement of help.

The methods used in this section are more complex than those used elsewhere in the book, therefore they are outlined more fully in this chapter. Results and their implications are discussed in subsequent subsections.

1. Methods

The analysis has two components. One is the comparison of the French cases with a group of the English cases chosen to be as similar as possible with respect to factors affecting the probability of admission to institutions for long-term care. The matching is the subject of section 1.1. The other analysis is based on statistical modelling. The dependent variable is whether the user is admitted to institutions for long-term care. That is the focus for the remainder of the methodological section. Section 1.2 describes the predictor variables and the effects hypothesised; section 1.3 the model form; and section 1.4, the modelling techniques. A further subsection reports the results, and a concluding subsection summarises the main results and discusses their implications.

1.1. Matching the English cases to the French sample to compare entry probabilities

A test of the first hypothesis requires the comparison of cases of similar needs. Therefore, a sample matching the French cases was drawn from the English database. The details are outlined in Table 30, which describes the matching process, and compares the groups used for the test of the difference between country samples in the probabilities of entry. A test of the significance of the difference between the matched group yields a significance level of .98, showing them to be practically identical. This strict matching entailed the loss of 20 French cases. There was therefore a sacrifice of representativeness in the French sample in order to gain greater comparability. In this France-focused research question, it was appropriate to give representativeness of the English

Table 30. Matching of English and French populations for comparison of entry to institutions

The three criteria adopted for the matching of the populations are: the user's disability level (using Isaacs and Neville disability indicators), the user's gender, and whether the user lives alone. Low disability cases (with no probability of getting ACTP) are excluded from the samples. This group matching process yields the following eight subcategories. The table below shows the final distribution of English and French samples used for the comparison of transition probabilities in the French and English cases.

Need interval disability level[a], *whether lives alone, sex*	*French sample*		*English sample*	
	No.	*%*	*No.*	*%*
Short, alone, female	15	17.6	15	17.4
Short, alone, male	13	15.3	18	20.9
Short, not alone, female	5	5.9	5	5.8
Short, not alone, male	2	2.4	2	2.3
Critical, alone, female	16	18.8	16	18.6
Critical, alone, male	20	23.5	15	17.4
Critical, not alone, female	13	15.3	14	16.3
Critical, not alone, male	1	1.2	1	1.2
Total	85		86	

Exact Pearson Chi-squared statistic: χ^2=1.552; Df=7; p=0.9809

[a] Disability level using categories from Isaacs and Neville (1975): critical, short, long, independent.

sample the lower priority.

For the modelling, precise matching is less important because the predictor variables include the one in which the two groups differ: disability. Therefore, a less strict matching criterion was used, increasing the representativeness of the British sample. Both French groups (and so both sets of matched English groups) were selected to cover only those with a level of disability at which a substantial proportion received ACTP, so that the persons involved could in principle apply for the benefit with reasonable probability of receiving it.

1.2. Predictors and postulated effects

The discussion is relevant only to the modelling undertaken to answer the second question. The indicators used in the final model for the French data are summarised in Table 31. Table 32 defines the variables used in the English modelling. Tables 33 and 34 provide a full listing of all variables considered in the modelling. Just the variable names are given. They are described fully on pages 205-207.

Policy variables: cash benefits

Levels of ACTP and attendance allowance were hypothesised to have a positive effect on the hours of formal and informal care, and negative direct and indirect effects on the probability of entry.[1]

The ACTP is the outcome of an allocation by the COTOREP at the level of the *département*, based on assessment by the staff of the *conseils généraux*. The assessments are based on national criteria. However, it is not obvious that the assessment methodology leads to allocations which precisely match the costs of providing services which will compensate equally for the disability: *'elle est attribuée de manière peu satisfaisante et sans garantie que son utilisation corresponde effectivement à des dépenses occasionnées par la dépendance'* (Commissariat général du plan, 1991, p.11). It is financed by the *départements*, whose levels of benefit vary greatly in generosity, reflecting policy priorities.

As in the case of ACTP, the aim of the attendance allowance is to provide a benefit for the more disabled: 'its purpose was, and remains, to help those among the disabled who require a considerable amount of personal attention' (Department of Health and Social Security, 1974, para. 37). During the period to which the English data relate, the main criteria for eligibility were either the need for continuous supervision to avoid danger to the beneficiary or others, or the need for frequent attention by day or prolonged attention by night for supervision or help with bodily functions (Bradshaw, 1988). However, its allocation is the outcome of a standardised medical assessment contracted by the Department of Social Security.

The English model also takes into account a negative subsidy: the

---

1 The collections did not allow comparisons of other benefits. Examples are service fees met by the *assistance sociale*, the level of invalid care allowance paid to the informal carers.

Table 31. Indicators used in the French model

Variable	*Mean*	*Sd*	*Min*	*Max*	*Q1*	*Md.*	*Q3*
ENTRY*	.21	.41	.00	1.00	.000	.000	.000
DISAB	6.04	2.02	3.36	9.76	4.357	5.171	8.536
ACTP	.08	.13	.00	.44	.000	.000	.221
CLOFEM*	.61	.49	.00	1.00	.000	1.000	1.000
INFMEAL	22.09	20.82	.00	84.00	.000	24.000	42.000
DISHOUS	43.85	81.48	.00	409.92	.000	.000	61.276
HIGHPCEXP*	.03	.17	.00	1.00	.000	.000	.000

* Dummy variable.

Table 32. Indicators used in the English model

Variable	*Mean*	*Sd*	*Min*	*Max*	*Q1*	*Md.*	*Q3*
ENTRY*		.09	.28	.00	1.00	.000	.000
CONFUSED*		.09	.28	.00	1.00	.000	.000
CAREANG*	.16	.37	.00	1.00	.000	.000	.000
COST		.00	.01	.00	.11	.000	.000
TIME2*		.49	.50	.00	1.00	.000	.000
DISAB		7.17	5.35	.00	17.80	2.426	6.391
MAL&ALO*	.10	.30	.00	1.00	.000	.000	.000
INCOME		2.68	1.29	1.00	10.00	2.000	2.000
INCOME2		8.84	10.44	1.00	100.00	4.000	4.000
INFHELP*	.54	.50	.00	1.00	.000	1.000	1.000
ALL&ANG	.00	.02	.00	.20	.000	.000	0.000

* Dummy variable.
Note that all the variables are described on pages 205-207.

Table 33. Other variables used in the French modelling

Variable	*Label*	*Mean*	*Sd*	*Min*	*Max*	*Q1*	*Md.*
HNO	1.05	1.42	.00	5.00	.000	.000	3.000
BEHAV*	1.27	1.07	.00	3.00	.000	1.000	2.000
WANDER*	.41	.49	.00	1.00	.000	.000	1.000
HOME*	.66	.48	.00	1.00	.000	1.000	1.000
SUITA*	.84	.37	.00	1.00	1.000	1.000	1.000
ISAAC	3.67	.47	3.00	4.00	3.000	4.000	4.000
INSERM	3.13	.71	1.00	4.00	3.000	3.000	4.000
AREA1*	.72	.45	.00	1.00	.000	1.000	1.000
MALE*	.37	.49	.00	1.00	.000	.000	1.000
MARRID*	.39	.49	.00	1.00	.000	.000	1.000
CIRC*	.31	.46	.00	1.00	.000	.000	1.000
RESP*	.07	.25	.00	1.00	.000	.000	.000
SKEL*	.45	.50	.00	1.00	.000	.000	1.000
CANC*	.06	.23	.00	1.00	.000	.000	.000
VIS*	.15	.36	.00	1.00	.000	.000	.000
ALZ*	.34	.47	.00	1.00	.000	.000	1.000
INCONT*	.47	.50	.00	1.00	.000	.000	1.000
BBOUND*	.11	.32	.00	1.00	.000	.000	.000
HBOUND*	.60	.49	.00	1.00	.000	1.000	1.000
INFPCT	18.64	24.35	.00	110.67	.000	11.667	27.500
SINF	14.11	15.41	.00	84.00	.000	12.000	20.000
HINF	11.82	19.60	.00	70.00	.000	.000	19.000
FORPCT	15.06	22.15	.00	98.00	.000	4.000	24.833
SFOR	2.27	6.12	.00	30.00	.000	.000	.000
AFOR	20.05	73.00	.00	466.20	.000	.000	.000
MFOR	8.23	14.80	.00	56.00	.000	.000	12.000
LIVCH*	.40	.49	.00	1.00	.000	.000	1.000
INFHOA*	.78	.42	.00	1.00	1.000	1.000	1.000

* Dummy variable.

Note that all the variables are described on pages 205-207.

Table 34. Other variables used in the English modelling

Variable	*Mean*	*Sd*	*Min*	*Max*	*Q1*	*Md.*	*Q3*
SINGLE*	.71	.45	.00	1.00	.000	1.000	1.000
BBOUND*	.01	.08	.00	1.00	.000	.000	.000
EPWANDER*	.01	.12	.00	1.00	.000	.000	.000
LOVEAFF*	.12	.32	.00	1.00	.000	.000	.000
MALE*	.27	.44	.00	1.00	.000	.000	1.000
CARMALE*	.14	.35	.00	1.00	.000	.000	.000
HHATTENT	0.74	.08	.00	.20	.000	.135	.135
ACOST2	8.28	9.72	.00	71.16	1.880	6.250	10.990
ACOST3	12.06	12.18	.00	91.40	4.443	7.975	15.550
FREQVSTS	4.06	2.08	.00	7.00	3.000	4.000	6.000
LONGVST	146.69	172.04	2.00	996.00	30.000	120.000	180.000
SSDHWORK*	.12	.32	.00	1.00	.000	.000	.000
SSDPCARE*	.02	.14	.00	1.00	.000	.000	.000
SSDMEALS*	.04	.19	.00	1.00	.000	.000	.000
SSDSHOPS*	.03	.17	.00	1.00	.000	.000	.000
SSDCMPNY*	.01	.10	.00	1.00	.000	.000	.000
HHRPENSN*	.20	.40	.00	1.00	.000	.000	.000
HBENEFIT*	.03	.17	.00	1.00	.000	.000	.000
CARAIDF*	.26	.95	.00	5.00	.000	.000	.000
EPAIDF*	.70	1.37	.00	4.00	.000	.000	1.000
TASKTIME	57.75	84.98	.00	480.	.000	22.50	85.000
ALLHTIME	35.65	82.17	.00	600.	.000	.000	30.000
ALLSTIME	50.43	96.99	.00	600.	.000	.000	60.000
RWDCARE*	.88	.32	.00	1.00	1.000	1.000	1.000
COTHPER*	.20	.40	.00	1.00	.000	.000	.000
CARHOSP*	.10	.30	.00	1.00	.000	.000	.000
HEATING*	.48	.50	.00	1.00	.000	.000	1.000
DEATHSP*	.04	.19	.00	1.00	.000	.000	.000
URIN*	.19	.40	.00	1.00	.000	.000	.000
FAECAL*	.08	.27	.00	1.00	.000	.000	.000
WALKAID*		.19	.40	.00	1.00	.000	.000
PET*	.14	.35	.00	1.00	.000	.000	.000

* Dummy variable.
Note that all the variables are described on pages 205-207.

amount of money paid in charges. Whereas a negative sign was hypothesised for attendance allowance and ACTP, a positive sign is hypothesised for the average charge payment. That effect has two components: an income effect and a substitution effect. The first is due to the reduction of income caused by paying the charges. This is the effect which is parallel to the attendance allowance effect. The second effect of charges paid is a substitution effect: their imposition makes home care more expensive in relation to residential care. Both effects would tend to increase the probability of admission.

Policy variables: hours of agency services

Hours of inputs were postulated to have a negative effect on entry probabilities; that is, marginal productivities were assumed to be positive. It is postulated that given need-related circumstances, hours of service reduce the probability of entry.

1.3. Control and intervening variables

Impairment, disability and handicap

It is hypothesised that disability level would have a positive effect on the probability of entry.

The principal indicators of disability covered the degree of difficulty in performing the five acts of daily living commonly the focus of American scaling and associated with personal care: mobility; incontinence; difficulties in performing instrumental activities of daily living; cognitive impairment developed during old age; and behaviour disturbance and problems associated with cognitive impairment and dementia-related diseases. Three general indicators were used in the exploratory modelling: interval need level, INSERM scale categories, and a (marginal) cost-weighted handicap score designed to be as highly correlated as possible with the costs of the formal care resources. The indicator is of what are called 'quasi-inputs' in the analytic framework of the 'production of welfare approach' (Davies and Challis, 1981, 1986; Davies and Knapp, 1981; Knapp, 1984). This, DISAB, emerged as the most significant disability-related predictor in the analysis. Indicators for each type of handicapping condition were also used.

Income support network and living arrangements
These include physical environment likely to exacerbate the handicapping effect's disabilities, and inputs of hours of care from each source of informal care for particular tasks.

Inputs were postulated to have positive marginal productivities; that is, negative effects on entry probabilities. Whether the elderly person lived alone or with others, the composition of the household was included because it was postulated (i) to affect the productivities of care inputs, and (ii) to indicate inputs which are discounted because respondents do not attribute the time to caring activities.

Disease types
The classification was not comprehensive even at a high level of generality. Neither did it differentiate the severity of the condition, or include prognostic information.

1.4. Methods and model form

Multivariate modelling techniques were used to search for, and estimate the magnitude of, the effects on the probabilities of service benefits in kind, and the (indirect) effects of cash benefits. The model form took account of the following:

- The substitute and complementary relations between formal and informal inputs for various tasks, allowing for relational propinquity for various tasks, as suggested by work on the substitution and hierarchy-compensatory hypotheses: in the USA, Cantor (1980) and Shanas (1979); in England, Qureshi and Walker (1989) and Qureshi (1990); and more partially in France, for which it has been suggested that elderly persons living alone are less likely to turn to their children for care (Le Disert et al., 1989, p.66). The definition of variables allowed for the possibility of the three types of causal process distinguished by Jette et al. (1995): 'substitution', 'buffering', and 'supplementation'.
- The possible non-monotonic effects of income and assets. Means would have (i) a *negative* effect among those of low income, and (ii) a *positive* effect among those who are better off. (i) At the lowest levels, there is little financial inducement to avoid entry, and housing is likely to be unsuitable, the local authority residential home offering better

amenities than ever before enjoyed. Therefore, entry to residential facilities would be more likely for the poorest than for the slightly better off. However, incentives change as the means reach the threshold for supplementary pension, and the income levels sufficient to pay residential home fees without spending down savings. At lower levels within this higher range, there would be greater uncertainty about whether they would be eligible for social security support in residential care.[2] With greater means, owner occupiers would have to dispose of their homes to pay for that residential care. Their homes would be more likely to be attractive and well-equipped, making residential care a less attractive option. So in this middle range of the distribution, the incentive to enter residential homes would have been much diminished. (ii) At higher levels, persons could retain much of their savings and pay for attractive residential care from income. Therefore, at this level of income one would anticipate that greater income might be associated with higher probabilities of admission than in the middle range of income.

1.5. Statistical techniques

The equations predicting admission were fitted using logistic regression analysis (Hosmer and Lemeshow, 1989). The model predicted entry between time i and time i+1, including among predictors risk factors at time i. There were two time intervals from the time of first use of the services, each of six months. The modelling sought simultaneity, it being hypothesised that the level of cash benefits might affect the utilisation of both agency services. Where found, the simultaneity was handled using 2SLS (Johnston, 1963).

2 The median price to the user of a place in a local authority old people's homes approximated £126 per week (1984/85 prices) in the sample; see Davies et al. (1990, Table A5.4).

2. Results

2.1. Average probability of entry

The French sample had an average probability of admission during the year of 23.5 per cent: twice as high as the English matched sample whose average probability was 11.6 per cent. The difference is significant at approximately the 2 per cent level with a one-tail test; $t=2.06$, $df=169$, $p=.0205$. That is unlikely to be due to the greater provision or higher standards of French accommodation.[3] It would seem that the French system is less effective at enabling persons to remain in their own homes.

2.2. Model coefficients

The results of the French model are described in Table 35 and Figure 3. The results of the English model are described in Table 36. The analyses yielded a final English model with only one equation.

The models for the French and English data both fit well, being significant at the .0000 level. The model for the French data throws more light on the part policy variables play in the causal processes.

The modelling for France revealed a more complex structure, in which the number of hours of care from agencies (principally *aide ménagère*) depends partly on the level of ACTP, and in which the number of hours of help from agencies with housework influences, and is influenced by, the input of help with meals from informal caregivers, all these variables

---

3 The OECD figures quoted in Chapter 1 show that the differences in the level of supply had closed by 1990. The difference in 1980 could have accounted for only a small fraction of the differences in the proportions discussed in the text. Standards of accommodation have not generally been thought to be high in French residential homes. Where there is a competitive market for residential care, near the northern French border with francophone Belgium, the flow is entirely from France to residential care in Belgium, with one estimate in 1990 (CODERPA du Nord) giving a figure of 25 per cent of all residential beds in the Belgium province of Hainaut being occupied by French citizens (Saunders, 1990). There is little evidence that this is due to differences in supply price, allowing for exchange rates.

Table 35. Results of the modelling of French provision

Predictor variables	*Dependent variables*							
	INFMEAL[a]		*DISHOUS*[b]		*ACTP*[a]		*ENTRY*[b]	
	Coef.	*P.*	*Coef.*	*P.*	*Coef.*	*P.*	*Coef.*	*P.*
DISHOUS	-.379	.014*					-.006	.059*
ACTP	58.606	.033*	154.543	.026			-10.253	.023*
DISAB	4.556	.021*	12.015	.004*	1.287	.019*	.434	.004*
INFMEAL			-2.637	.028			-.037	.011*
CLOSFEM							-1.390	.013*
HIGHPCEXP							4.456	.038*
Goodness of fit							.857[c]	.000[d]
R^2	.057		.126		.041			
Adj. R^2	.029		.099		.032			
Sig. (F test)	.112		.003		.037			

* one tail test.
[a]Estimated with two stage least squares procedure.
[b]Estimated with a logistic regression.
[c]Overall accuracy of prediction.
[d]Significance (Chi-square).

Table 36. Results of the modelling of English provision

	ENTRY[a]	
	Coef.	*P.*
CONFUSED	2.278	.000
COST	39.735	.006
TIME2	2.566	.000
CAREANG	1.862	.000*
DISAB	.046	.078*
MAL&ALO	1.019	.017*
INCOME	-1.104	.003
INCOME2	.104	.015
INFHELP	-.989	.011*
ALL&ANG	-23.341	.009
Goodness of fit	.92[b]	.000[c]

* one tail test.
[a] Estimated with a logistic regression.
[b] Overall accuracy of prediction.
[c] Significance (Chi-square).
Note that all the variables are described on pages 205-207.

Figure 3. Effects on entry of inputs of housework and ACTP. Direction and significance of relationships in the modelling of the probability of admission in the French sample

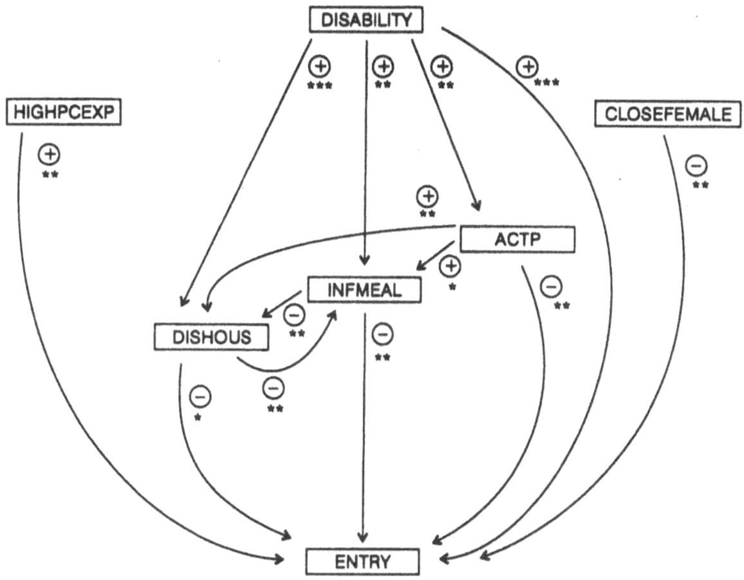

Significance levels: *** p < .01
** p < .05
* p < .10

being influenced by the disability of users. With respect to *policy variables*, the main features are:

• The modelling strongly suggests that ACTP reduces the probability of entry. The evidence about the effects of attendance allowance is more ambiguous.

The modelling for the French data revealed both direct and indirect effects of ACTP. The indirect effects are complicated by the interdependence of the number of hours of informal help with meals, and the number of formal hours of help with housework provided by agencies. ACTP has positive effects on the input of informal help with meals: p=.033 with a two-tail test (a two-tail test, because a coefficient with the opposite sign would have been compatible with the use of the ACTP more to enable the substitution of formal for informal care than for paying for more formal care). ACTP in addition to the existing informal input has a positive effect on informal inputs with meals, the effect being positively correlated with the degree of disability (p=.03 for a two-tail test, for an analogous reason), and also with inputs of housework among the more disabled (DISHOUS; p=.026). The direct effect of ACTP on reducing probability of entry is also significant: p=.0228 with a one-tail test.

An English sample which includes those whose disability is too low to have had a high probability of receiving ACTP in France, but with nevertheless a probability of receiving attendance allowance in England, suggests that attendance allowance too has the predicted effect, but only for some recipients. The recipients for whom it seems to have the effect are those whose principal informal caregivers experienced feelings of anger because of the caring. The effect is significant at the 1 per cent level with a two-tail test. Perhaps attendance allowance provides a financial incentive to carers which offsets the effect of the feelings of anger on the probability that the user will enter a residential institution.

The English data also allow the estimation of the effect of the charge to — that is, copayment by — users (COST). For the sample of 588, COST has a highly significant entry-increasing effect on the probability of entry (p=.003 with a one-tail test), given the additive effect of two indicators of disability: level of disability (DISAB), and whether confused (CONF).

• Hours of help with housework from agencies has the predicted direct effect on the probability of entry in the French sample to an increasing degree with higher disability: p=.0592, with a one-tail test. This is a buffering effect (Jette et al., 1995; Davies et al., 1995). There is no sign that agency housework has a comparable effect for the English sample, as has been found in other analyses, despite the greater likelihood of those obtaining higher levels of care claiming that, but for the services received, they would be unable to continue to live independently in their own homes (Davies et al., 1990; Davies and Baines, 1994).

3. Control variables

Disability

In the French sample, it appears that disability, measured by DISAB, has both direct and a complex of indirect effects. The direct effect is strong and in the predicted direction: p=.00415 for a one-tail test. However, the indirect effects are negative.

In the English sample, predictors include general disability (DISAB) on the one hand, and confusion on the other. The literature has repeatedly shown how cognitive impairment associated with behavioural disturbance precipitates entry to institution. Again, the effects are well-determined in this sample. However, in the English model, the expression of anger by the carer with their caring role is a strong predictor of the probability of entry (p=.000), as it is in some other British modelling (Davies and Baines, 1994).

Informal care

Informal care has a predictably important influence. In the French model, the presence of a close female relation living in the same household has a major effect (p=.0127 with one-tail test). Informal inputs with meals also has a clear effect.

In the English model, INFHELP, MAL&ALO, and CAREANG have powerful additive effects. The buffering effect of attendance allowance on those with carers having feelings of anger has already been mentioned. CAREANG no doubt captures stress, the history of relationships, the degree to which the nature of the care required offends norms and expectations of the caring obligations of persons of that degree of relational propinquity, and the other factors well described by sociologists and gerontologists. Other English analyses have found a wider variety of effects of informal care on the probability of entry (Davies et al., 1990; Davies and Baines, 1994).

In neither sample was there evidence of the 'supplementation effect' postulated by Jette et al. (1995). Jette et al. themselves did not find such an effect in their study in Massachusetts.

Income

The model for English data shows the importance of income. The results for the income terms precisely fit the above argument about the incentive effects at different income levels. The combined effect of the two income terms makes the relationship non-monotonic. The values of the coefficients yield a minimum value of the probability of entry at £126 per week (1984/85 prices), approximately the full cost of a place in a local authority home. It is an income which was 3.5 times the level of the state weekly pension for single pensioners aged 80 and over (64 per cent of the English sample lived alone). The official poverty line, the supplementary benefit level, was little different from the pension level. Therefore the minimum value was at a level which was considerably above the official poverty level.

3.1. *The principal results*

In France, both a form of service in kind from home care agencies and the ACTP appeared to have an effect on probabilities, the level of ACTP affecting probabilities indirectly, through its influence on the receipt of agency help with housework, as well as directly; but the direct ACTP effect is clearer and stronger. Provision is made to check that recipients of ACTP use the benefits to procure care from others. There are *associations mandataires* to assist persons to use ACTP to procure help. And, indeed, that ACTP was used to procure service from others by direct employment, to encourage informal or quasi-informal helpers, as well as to help to meet the general costs of disability, is compatible with the results of other research which has found that the ACTP is in fact used to compensate a third person for care: *'les motifs compatibles avec l'allocation compensatrice: vouloir rémunérer la tierce personne'* (Arfeux-Vaucher, 1986, pp.85,86). Of course, it remains valid to argue that the allocation of ACTP could be still more precisely tuned (Commissariat général du plan, 1991). Indeed, Figure 1 in Chapter 1 illustrates some anomalies in the association between receipt and disability level.

In England, attendance allowance but not indicators of formal service input had an effect on probabilities for some users only. That result was confirmed by other analyses of the same databases (Davies et al., 1990; Davies and Baines, 1994). The earlier analysis discovered that the marginal productivities of home care services for a range of less ambiguous outcomes seemed generally to be too low to be detected in the presence of the noise caused by specification and measurement errors.

3.2. Conclusions

Marginal productivities

The British critique established that the improvement of equity and efficiency required the improvement of the marginal productivities of inputs in terms of outcomes of evaluative significance. Though productivities depend partly on targeting, the improvement of targeting in itself would be insufficient. The results for the UK again illustrate the low marginal productivities prior to the reform. Their improvement would require both better brokerage and changes in the nature and content of the services themselves.

Putting forward a tougher analysis of weaknesses in supply and its coordination, the Schopflin report started to correct an imbalance in French policy analysis. The projects of Mme Weil, Health Minister in the Balladur government, illustrate that this new emphasis was taken seriously in the development of the proposed *prestation autonomie*. From this perspective, the *prestation spécifique dépendance* is slightly disappointing. As we shall see, and as has been illustrated in the experiment in the Département de l'Aine, it would be compatible with the care management integration of inputs which could raise the marginal productivities of services, but the new *prestation* does not require this. The low marginal productivities of service inputs show that the new emphasis is needed in France as in the UK. France has something to learn from experience overseas in the design of general models and the adapatation of the artefacts developed for coordinated, flexible and user-responsive care whose resource allocations take account of cost-effectiveness in the use of public funds at all levels.

Modal choice at the individual level

To British commentators now accustomed to the logic of the community care reforms, particularly visible is that the financers and brokers of care in France have no incentives to weigh up the relative costs and benefits for the individual of alternative residential and home care modes, and to seek to influence choices accordingly.

Indeed, giving an interesting twist to the development of studies of the relative costs of residential and home care modes, one of the biggest and best of the international studies produced estimates that when account is taken of the value of the time given to caring by informal carers, the care (including health care) costs were higher for persons living in private households than in the main forms of institutions other than long-stay hospitals, *'long séjour'* (Bouget et al., 1990, Table 3-26). The confidence intervals suggested significant differences at all disability levels between costs at home and in residential homes with the medical supervision of some beds (*'maisons de retraite avec sections de cure medicale'*). The results were in conflict with the assumption that there was a range of dependency within which one mode of care would be more costly than a second, but other ranges at which the second mode would be the less costly. If valid, the argument would have the important implication that the shift in the balance of provision towards home care would be costly. Therefore, it would be necessary to ensure that home care resources were used most effectively. It would be important to engage in the long war of attrition accompanied by political and professional battles necessary to improve the effectiveness of the system in creating and coordinating inputs.

However, it would be fallacious to argue that the more desired home care is always more costly than facility care, even if the estimates in Bouget et al. were broadly correct.[4] First, what matters is the cost of benefits valued in their own right, not the cost associated with varying levels of dependency in modes of care likely to produce quite different qualities of life and care for the elderly persons themselves and their families. The French study does not take into account variations between modes in these qualities of life and care. Secondly, it is not the average cost given dependency which is important for making the best use of modes of care in modern community care. The appropriate selection

4 The valuation of the time of informal carers is inevitably controvertible. But, being based on mean income per hour, costs of home care are more sensitive to the assumption than other forms of care. The costs of informal care were estimated on average to be 58.4 per cent of the total care costs. An appended table shows the costs of informal care as a proportion of the total costs of care, based on the estimates in Bouget et al. (1990, Tables 3-8). Discounting the costs of informal care altogether would yield total care costs for persons at home only non-significantly higher than of persons in residential homes.

of mode of care is most important when costs would be high and outcomes poor in one mode, but low and high respectively in the other. In such cases, it is the fact that different factors make costs and outcomes high and low in the various modes of care which makes the best choice of mode important, as the Kent Community Care Project and its replications and extensions have shown (Davies and Challis, 1986; Challis et al., 1991, 1994; Davies and Chesterman, 1998). The traditional argument has oversimplified this. The identification of these circumstances requires the matching of resources to the needs of individuals in the form of help in the choice of care mode, as well as the packaging of resources and the formulation of strategies for individuals within care modes. The Schopflin proposal for handling the *prestation dépendance* goes some way towards securing the necessary matching of resources to needs, the benefit being based on assessments by a multidisciplinary team (Commissariat général du plan, 1991).

Cash and care

The results throw new light on the potential advantages of the emphasis on cash payments as a means of procuring care in countries building from Bismarckian social insurance systems. The priority which Chirac has given to the new *prestation* from the time of the election campaign onwards, and his justification of it in terms of making it possible to stay at home rather than enter institutions as well as employment generation, suggests that there was never a real danger of its subversion in France, despite the number of cross-currents introduced by interest-group proposals and pressure. No doubt the introduction of the *prestation spécifique dépendance*, designed to provide a capped top-up to ACTP rather than a benefit based more on the German reform, was mainly due to the need to meet the conditions for joining the single European currency and facing the economic consequences of doing so. There may have been a wish to put in place financing mechanism which would change the incentive structures facing conservative providers who were insufficiently sensitive to the needs for changing their service patterns, the new arrangements increasing the probability of targeting on those of greater dependence, and encouraging recipients to use the benefit in ways which secured most benefit for the cost. In this, the French strategy reflects the new emphasis on incentives rather than political persuasion, or the traditional command-control techniques of public administration as a means of implementing policy change (Davies and Challis, 1986; Kraan et al., 1991; Baldock and Evers, 1992; Davies, 1993), as well as an emphasis on the regulation of the system through demand rather than supply. However, it will be important to monitor how well it achieves this objective with research using methodologies which are not generally applied to community and long-term care in France.

For the UK, the results support a general proposition akin to the issue of the marginal productivities of services in kind raised in Davies et al. (1990). We should focus on making the important cash benefits for community care more effective in extending the choice of receiving care in their own homes: in effect, raise the marginal productivity of attendance allowance with respect to one of the most important goals of community care policy.

In the short term, we have to work with the productivities which exist. An immediate issue should be the balance between expenditure on a cash benefit for the procurement of care, and direct expenditure on the formal services by the financing agency. In France, what would be the effects on the probability of admission of increases in the level of the two kinds of input: ACTP and agency inputs for housework? In England, what would be the effects of increased levels of attendance allowance and of decreased levels of charges? The next section presents estimates of the implications of our productivity estimates.

3.3. *Effects of varying provision levels on entry*

Consider a model with two forms of provision: home care and residential care. Assume (i) that the duration of utilisation of one or other service is not affected by the proportion of time spent in each; (ii) that, once having been admitted to residential care, no one is discharged to home care; and (iii) there are no deaths or other exits from the two systems during the period. Then, given that there are ranges of home care spending at which the expenditure is less than the price of the period in an institution, there might be a decrease in the total cost incurred given an increase in ACTP or housework hours from formal agencies (in France) or an increase in attendance allowance in England (Greene et al., 1993). If that is so, there would be negative partial derivatives of total cost with respect to the cost of the benefit in question. The proposition is explained in Table 37.

Table 37 shows that in the French sample the partial derivatives are negative for most of the sample for each form of input. So more expenditure either on agency inputs for housework or on ACTP would reduce costs for most cases. However, dTC/dC_{ACTP} has much higher negative values for 74 per cent of the sample than has dTC/dC_{HFOR} for any of the sample.

How much effect the model suggests would be achieved by various increases in ATCP and housework hours can be read off from Figures 4 and 5. (i) The comparisons are made for persons at three levels of DISAB. (The model finds that the effects depend on the level of DISAB.) (ii) For persons at each level, there are two curves. They both start from the current level of probability of admission. One curve shows the effects of varying increases in ACTP. The other shows the effects of increases in housework hours from the agencies. (iii) Figure 4 assumes the inputs of time by informal carers in meals-related help to be unrelated to ACTP and agency housework hours; that is, it ignores the interdependence shown in Figure 3, and Figure 5 takes account of that interdependence, and illustrates how the simultaneity reflects (i) the substitution of agency-provided housework for informal help with meals, and (ii) the positive effect of ACTP on informal help with meals. The first swamps the direct effects of housework on the probabilities, but show they are in turn swamped by the direct effects at higher levels of input. The differences between the corresponding curves in the two diagrams indicates the impact of the effect of the interdependence between ACTP and DISHOUS on informal help with meals.

The results from the English effect did not find that service levels influenced entry probabilities. However, attendance allowance was found to have an effect for some users: those whose carers felt angry towards users. Figure 6 illustrates the strength of the effect. The curve may be compared with those in Figure 5.

3.4. Discussion

The general conclusion is that it may be feasible for the cash benefits to achieve some of the sophistication of community care policy of

Table 37. The marginal effect of ACTP and agency housework inputs on total cost

The table shows the partial derivatives of total cost with respect to the cost of the input in question. Negative values in the partial derivatives reveal scope for long-term savings by increasing the levels of inputs for a particular policy variable. The more negative the value, the greater the scope for savings.

Changes in total expenditures associated with marginal additional expenditure on ACTP and direct expenditure on housework provided by agencies in France:

Input	$\partial TC/\partial C_{INPUT}$	%	*Cum. %*
Direct expenditure on agency-provided housework	-15 to -10	9.6	9.6
	-10 to - 5	28.8	38.4
	-5 to -2.5	23.9	62.3
	-2.5 to 0	22.6	84.9
	0 to 2.5	15.1	100.0
Expenditure on ACTP	-130 to -80	16.4	16.4
	-80 to -40	29.5	45.9
	-40 to -15	28.1	74.0
	-15 to -10	7.5	81.5
	-10 to -5	4.8	86.3
	-5 to 0	10.3	96.6
	0 to 5	3.4	100.0

Table 37 continued

The calculations are based on a model which focuses on the effect of total expenditure of additional expenditure on ACTP and Housework formal help. The model hypothesises long-term care costs to be the average between the residential care costs and home care costs, weighted by the probability of going into residential care and staying in the community respectively. Mathematically this can be restated as:

$$LTC=\alpha_r{*}C_r+(1+ar){*}C_h$$

with LTC being the long-term care cost, α_r, the probability of going into residential care, C_r being the cost of residential care, and C_h the cost of home help. Therefore, given our logit modelling, the probability of entry into residential care can be stated as:

Prob. =

$$\frac{1}{1+W} \text{ with } \Omega=e^{-(.4343*disab-10.2530*actp-.0367*infmeal-1.390*clofem-.0064*dishous+4.4559*hipcexp-2.1190)}$$

where e is the base of the natural logarithm.

We can now estimate the long-term care cost per client by applying the first of the formulae described above, and applying to this the partial derivative of the long-term cost for changes in both HFOR and ACTP. The final formulae giving the marginal returns for changes in expenditures on services (housework and ACTP) are:

For HFOR: $\frac{\partial LTC}{\partial HFOR}=(C_r-C_h){*}\frac{\partial Prob}{\partial HFOR}+(1-Prob)$

For ACTP: $\frac{\partial LTC}{\partial ACTP}=(C_r-C_h){*}\frac{\partial Prob.}{\partial ACTP}+(1-Prob.)$

Only if the estimated value of such equations is negative can we expect some savings to arise because of an increase in the provision of home help. If this happens, the direct increase in cost due to the input of further home help will be offset by long-term savings due to a reduction in the probability of using the service with higher unit costs: residential care. Consequently, the more negative the value, the greater the scope for savings.

Figure 4. Probability of entry to residential institutions with varying levels of ACTP and agency housework: not allowing for the dependence of informal inputs into meals provision in response to ACTP and agency housework, for users at three disability levels

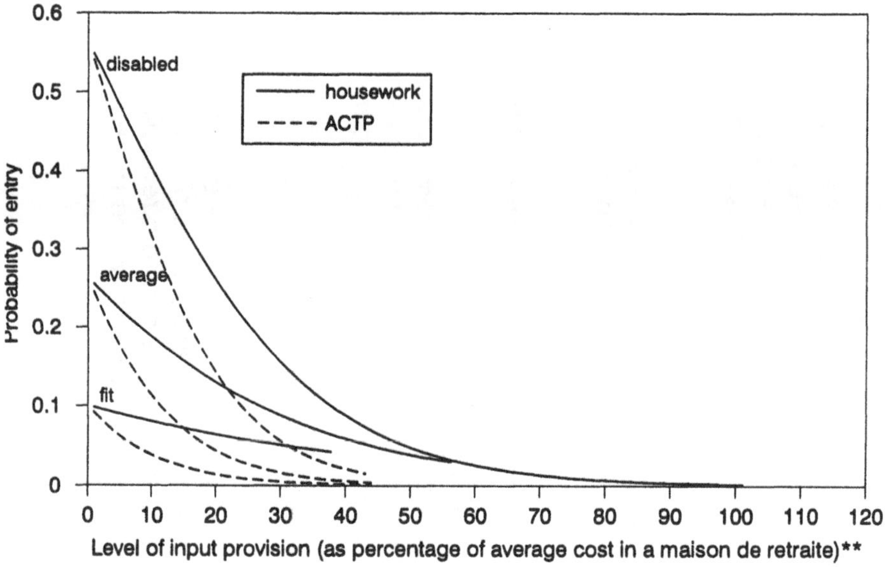

The curves are plotted at three levels of disability: 'disabled' (maximum level in the sample); 'average' (mean); and 'fit' (minimum level in the sample).

* Because the curves are plotted independently of one another, one cannot read off the optimal mix of the two inputs from the diagram.

** The upper limit shown is within the range observed in the sample.

services in kind. In the UK, the number of aged recipients of attendance allowances has been rising quickly, as has expenditure.[5] Increasingly,

5 Expenditure on attendance allowance in FY1993 was 8.9 times higher than in 1979; 1.54 times higher than in 1989; and the number of recipients aged 85 and over was 8.9 times higher than the number in 1979, and 1.8 times the number in 1989 (Department of Social Security, 1993).

Figure 5. Probability of entry to residential institutions with varying levels of ACTP and agency housework: allowing for the dependence of informal inputs into meals provision in response to ACTP and agency housework, for users at three disability levels

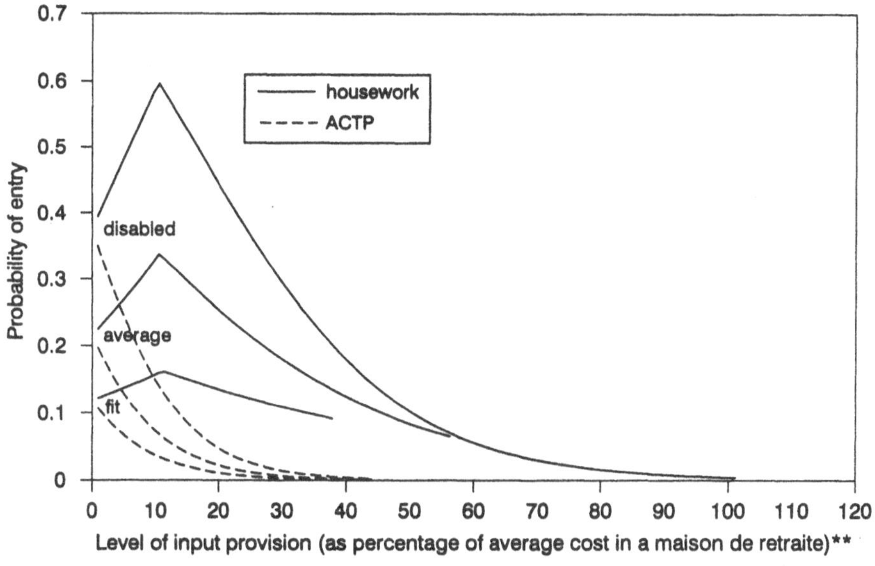

The curves are plotted at three levels of disability: 'disabled' (maximum level in the sample); 'average' (mean); and 'fit' (minimum level in the sample).
* Because the curves are plotted independently of one another, one cannot read off the optimal mix of the two inputs from the diagram.
** The upper limit shown is within the range observed in the sample.

the benefit has been used by local authorities to create the income from which user charges could be met. However, assessment criteria and the crudeness of the benefit structure does not tune the benefit received to the probable costs of meeting needs. Though itself crude, the ACTP is more successful in these respects. The effectiveness of attendance allowances could also be improved by providing recipients with access to brokerage support subsequent to assessment. This could be optional for some, compulsory for others.[6]

6 We observe that the French complain about the delays and diminished

Figure 6. Probability of entry to residential institutions with varying levels of attendance allowance, for cases in which the informal helper is angry (CAREANG)

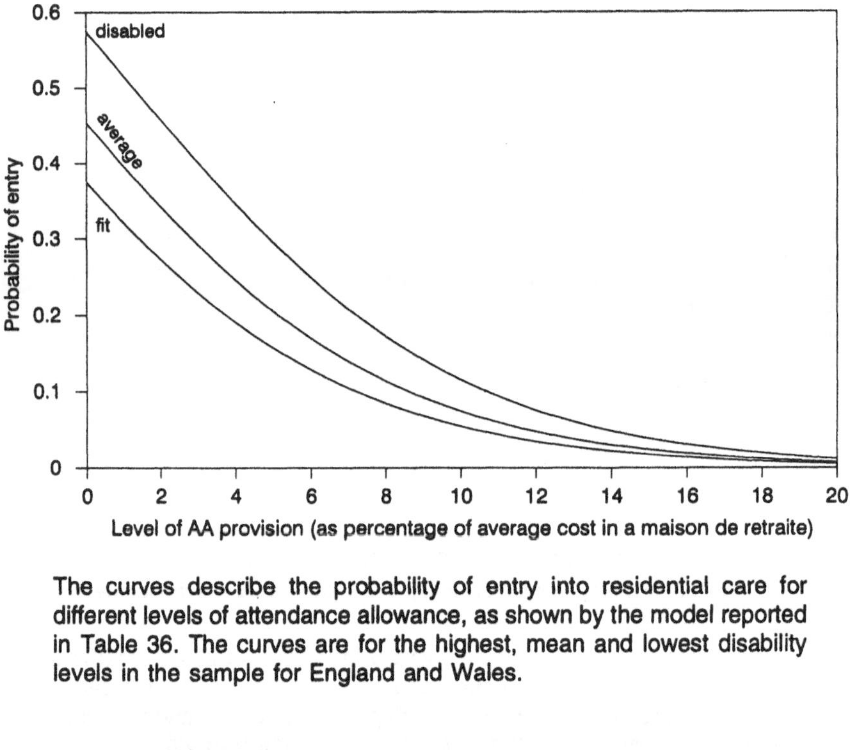

The curves describe the probability of entry into residential care for different levels of attendance allowance, as shown by the model reported in Table 36. The curves are for the highest, mean and lowest disability levels in the sample for England and Wales.

---

impact of care in allocation decisions, because the *départemental* COTOREPS are distant, at the level of a large county. That is reminiscent of American experience. The rigidity of American targeting and case management is partly the result of a similar separation. So it is arguable that the role of the care management team should be extended to allocating cash allowances for those for when there is an imperative directly to purchase formal services, as in Michigan (Linsk et al., 1992). In that way, we would make more use of the resources and avoid heavy transaction costs. The arrangement might have another advantage. Linsk et al. (1992) show that the attitudes of the policy-makers to the subsidisation of family carers were less dominated by the fear of cost escalation in Michigan's Adult Home Help programme, in which state employees negotiate the individual allocations with the elderly persons, than in the Illinois Community Care Program, in which state

Such a benefit could help to improve effectiveness and efficiency in the real economy of care. It would create incentives to users to compensate for dependence in performing daily living tasks by finding flexible ways of securing care and support, sometimes combining material as well as human inputs. Doing that, it could contribute towards the integration of informal, quasi-informal and formal care. It could also contribute towards the empowerment and integration of elderly people, while reinforcing social solidarity and communitarian means and values more generally. Since these are clearly aims of the *préstation spécifique dépendance*, how it works will deserve close study.

This at least partial reintegration of a cash benefit with the procedures for brokering services in kind would be the extension of one of the main principles which has been applied in community care reform: consolidating the responsibility for balancing the marginal benefits of additional expenditures on alternative means in one politically accountable agency, and within it, in one manager at each level of territorial aggregation. It would amount to creating special arrangements for some groups who are particularly at risk, with boundaries of financing responsibility differently drawn from those for the population in general.

It would be important to evaluate other costs and benefits. In doing so, it might well emerge that divisions of labour should be redrawn in other respects also. For instance, there are now much greater gains from medical interventions for frail elderly persons than existed when the present divisions of responsibility were established. Also, the price of acute hospital treatment has risen massively in relation to that of the low-tech personal social care for which it creates needs and demands. Therefore, the implications of the argument for the redivision of labour might well imply the development of models integrating financing and supply brokerage, and covering the whole range of health as well as

financing is channelled through non-governmental organisations, and where, therefore, the individual allocation decisions are not directly made by state employees. In the UK, the scope of the jurisdiction of the command-control economy in the financing, brokerage, and the implementation of trade and industry policies for the persons of low income, with its direct organisational authority and accountability, as distinct from the market, may contribute to balancing the promise of flexibility against the fear of escalating public expenditure.

community care, as is attempted in some American models whose relevance for the UK is worth exploration (Davies, 1994; Davies and Baines, 1994).

There are various reasons why the basic evaluative criterion used in this section — the reduction in the probability of admission to institutions for long-term care — is likely to become less relevant: among others, changes in the physical and social environments of facilities, the development of a wider range of facilities and arrangements by which handicapped persons can receive what the Anglo-Saxons call 'shelter-with-care', new more flexible methods of providing home care in ways which can help to make the utilisation of shelter-with-care for short episodes for providing respite to informal caregivers, mixing social care with assessment, rehabilitation and sub-acute treatment in a career in which the longest periods are spent at home. The trends were already visible by the mid-eighties. Some then argued that, for such reasons, the evaluative criteria should increasingly become lifetime costs and benefits, not short-term costs and benefits (Davies and Challis, 1986). That must be the subject of a later cross-national study.

Appendix table to Chapter 7. Imputed costs of informal care as a proportion of total expenditure on dependency-related services and informal care costs 1988

	Dependency level							
	1	2	3	4	5	6	7	Overall
Imputed value of informal help/ percentage of total care costs (per cent)	74.8	54.9	51.8	37.2	67.7	64.0	62.9	58.4

Source: Bouget et al., 1990, Table 3-8, p.136.

1 = None, 2 = Very slight, 3 = Slight, 4 = Average, 5 = High, 6 = Very high, 7 = Extreme

The imputation of informal care costs was decribed in Bouget et al. (1990, pp.367-72). Expenditures on formal services were for privately employed home care (*gardes malades* or *femmes de ménage*), home help (*aide ménagère*), and personal care assistants (*soins à domicile*).

Part III

8 Discussion

The study has (i) compared the structures for the publicly-subsidised supply of community services for elderly persons in France and England, and (ii) described the need-related circumstances of those receiving different quantities of service, and changes in the need-related circumstances and support inputs over time. The comparison has revealed important features which should be of interest to policy-makers and managers in each country.

One way in which we hope that it will prove useful is for its treatment of the main themes:

- persons in what need-related circumstances obtain how much of what type of service, and with what effect on their probabilities of being able to continue living in the community rather than entering institutions for long-term care;
- informal and formal caregiving; and
- cash payments to pay for care rather than the subsidisation of care in kind.

A second way is the provision of general evidence which is usually comparable for the two countries for others to use around their own interests, and the publication of findings of general interest.

1. Summary of main findings

1.1. The evidence as a source

How few comparable but detailed data there are for community care in the two countries has become clear in this investigation and our collaboration with a team from the *Centre pluridisciplinaire sur vieillissement* on the comparison of equity and efficiency argument in the British and French literatures. Indeed, this modest study appears to be the largest, most rigorous and most detailed comparative collection. For this reason, we have included more tabular evidence than has been strictly necessary for the foci of our argument — just as we have included more description of the recent history of English and French policy-making, because much of the material would be inaccessible to many readers and could be collated only with great effort. Readers principally interested in the need-related circumstances of users would turn to Chapter 5. Others would turn to Chapters 6 and 7 if their main interests were in how agencies complement and supplement the activities of family and what the Anglo-Saxons call 'informal caregivers', where the interest is the comparison of a system in which the *obligation alimentaire still holds sway, with a system without it.*

1.2. Comparisons between England and France

These comparisons are based on the samples of recipients of a defined set of home and community services in three pairs of areas, each pair consisting of an English and a French area matched by social and environmental circumstances.

Need-related circumstances: users

- The proportion in the highest interval need category,[1] 'critical interval need', was higher in the French than in the English areas: 62.9 per cent compared with 27.7 per cent.
- A similar proportion was able to perform personal care tasks: 93.5 per cent in England, 94.4 per cent in France.
- A higher proportion was able to perform household activities in England: 43.5 per cent compared with 26.0 per cent.
- The proportion reporting urinary incontinence was slightly higher in England: 24.7 per cent compared with 17.5 per cent.
- Similar proportions were aged 75 or over: 68.9 per cent in England, compared to 70.6 per cent in France. Within that age range, however, there was a lower proportion in England of those aged 85 or over: 14.3 per cent compared to 29.4 per cent.
- A higher proportion was married or living with a partner in England: 52.8 per cent compared to 32.9 per cent.
- The proportion of users or their spouse or partner who were home

1 Interval need categories are defined in Chapter 4.

owners was higher in France: 72.7 per cent compared with 50.7 per cent.

- The proportion with access to an inside toilet was higher in England: 97.1 per cent compared with 89.3 per cent in France.

Help from 'informal caregivers'

- The proportion of users who received help from a close relative was lower in England than in France: 12.5 per cent compared with 43.9 per cent.
- The proportion of users who received help from non-relatives was lower in England than in France: 2.8 per cent compared with 16.7 per cent.
- There was also a lower percentage of users in England who received informal help for any task: 38.6 per cent compared with 51.8 per cent.

Formal agency response to need

- The percentage of users who had received formal help with any task at the time of the first assessment was lower in England than in France: 42.1 per cent compared with 73.6 per cent.
- Similarly, there was a lower proportion of users in England who had received formal help for personal care tasks by the time of the first assessment: 33.5 per cent as opposed to 51.0 per cent in France.
- However, the percentage of users who had received formal help with meals by the time of the first assessment was higher in England: 34.3 per cent compared with 20.7 per cent.
- For help with shopping, the proportion of users in the English sample was also higher as at the time of the first assessment: 34.3 per cent compared with 23.7 per cent for the French sample.

Substitution between formal and informal inputs

- The analysis looked for patterns of substitution between formal and informal services. It was hypothesised that informal carers would de- crease their involvement in response to an increase in the level of formal service input. However, the data did not offer any strong evidence to support this; for all tasks and over all periods of time, only 12.4 per cent of cases showed any degree of reduction in the level of informal help subsequent to an increase in the level of formal inputs.

• The analysis looked for patterns of substitution between formal and informal services. It was hypothesised that informal carers would decrease their involvement in response to an increase in the level of formal service input. However, the data did not offer any strong evidence to support this; for all tasks and over all periods of time, only 12.4 per cent of cases showed any degree of reduction in the level of informal help subsequent to an increase in the level of formal inputs.

• There is evidence that the proportion of cases showing some substitution of formal for informal care inputs does increase over time, but the figures are small.

• The main task for which there is evidence of substitution between formal and informal care inputs is for personal care tasks, such as washing, toileting or bathing.

The probabilities of entry into institutions for long-term care

• When matched with respect to key factors affecting the probability of entry into institutional care, the French sample presented an average rate of admission twice as high as for the English matched sample.

• However, the results of statistical modelling showed that the French formal service inputs had a greater impact than the equivalent English services in reducing the probability of entry into institutional care.

• In both the French and English samples, cash benefits were found to be more effective than formal services in reducing the probability of entry into institutional care, although in the case of the English attendance allowance, this effect was much more limited than was the case for the French *allocation compensatrice* (ACTP).

• For the French sample, although both formal services and cash allowance showed a positive effect in reducing the probability of entry into institutional care, the effect was much more marked in the case of the cash allowance, ACTP.

• There is evidence that, for the French sample, there could be potential for savings in the long-term care costs to be derived from increases in the provision of home care services, and particularly ACTP, as a result of the likely reduction in the probability of demand for entry into more expensive, shelter-with-care modes.

1.3. Comparisons between the three French areas

The three French areas for which the data were collected were Athis Mons, La Manche and St Omer.

Athis Mons is a suburb of Paris, near Orly airport in the *département* of Essonne (91). Its population is mainly metropolitan French in origin and works principally in white-collar and middle-class jobs. An important feature of the service system was a team who provided a single point of entry to services, both domiciliary and shelter-with-care, through a *service de coordination*. This team had been set up with the help of project money from, among other agencies, the Fondation de France and the *Caisse régionale d'assurance maladie* and was considered to be a good model of coordination, particularly for home care, with co-located not-for-profit associations providing both home help and personal care through both a *service de soins à domicile* and a personal care service of *garde à domicile.*

La Manche (50) is the Normandy *département* which includes the Cherbourg peninsular, and is characterised by some important industrial sites such as ship-building and nuclear power, but with a considerable rural area focused on dairy products, and hence with a relatively static population with close local family links. The service system which formed the second site for the French study was the *Service départemental d'action social,* the local authority social work team. The policy in La Manche was actively to favour the use of the cash allowance ACTP, in preference to *aide sociale,* to pay for domiciliary care for elderly people. In the view of the *conseil général,* this had the advantage that the users would be able to buy more hours of home care through *associations mandataire* than the *département* itself could purchase using the official home care organisations at the full hourly rate for such service.[2]

St Omer is a medium-sized town in the Pas de Calais (62). It is in the former mining area that once covered much of northern France. Some evidence of this can be seen in the sample data on, say, the percentage of users who are widowed, reflecting the early deaths suffered by former miners, and the high proportion of owner-occupiers, since the former mining concerns had a policy of selling off their housing stock to the existing tenants. The service delivery in St Omer was of

2 This is examined in full in Chapter 3.

the unified home help and nursing care type, provided by one co-located not-for profit *Association d'aide et soins à domicile.*

The data are examined in more detail in the Annex, but some of the more significant comparisons between the three sites are highlighted here. One of the features illustrated by the summary findings presented below is the difference between La Manche and the other sites. In La Manche our focus was the *aide sociale* and the ACTP; that is, the most politically controlled of the forms of obligatorily and public policy-centred funding entitlements. It was broader elsewhere. The significance is its contribution to understanding how with one set of arrangements a mixed system of social insurance and social assistance funding worked.

Need-related circumstances of users

- The highest percentage of most dependent users in the critical interval need category at the time of the first assessment was in La Manche: 72.5 per cent, compared with Athis Mons (54.8 per cent) and St Omer (54.5 per cent).
- Across all three sites, the percentage of users in the critical interval need category at the time of the first assessment was 62.9 per cent. By the time of the second assessment, of those users still at home and receiving help, 60.0 per cent were in the critical interval need category, and at the time of the third assessment this was 54.4 per cent.

Informal help

- The lowest percentage of users who were married or living with a partner at the time of the first assessment was in Athis Mons, at 21.3 per cent, with St Omer at 25.0 per cent and La Manche at 48.4 per cent.
- The highest percentage of users still receiving informal help with any task at the time of the second assessment was in La Manche, at 96.1 per cent, compared with 81.3 per cent in Athis Mons and 37 per cent in St Omer.
- By the time of the third assessment, for La Manche the percentage was 91.9 per cent, with 72 per cent in Athis Mons and 29.4 per cent of users in St Omer.
- At the second assessment, the average number of hours given by informal carers to help users with any task was 412.5 per month across all three areas. St Omer showed a higher figure, of 612.8 hours per

month; La Manche had an average figure of 433.4 hours and Athis Mons 296.1 hours per month for informal care with any task.[3]

• By the time of the third assessment, the average for the number of hours users received from informal caregivers for help with any task had fallen slightly to 364.7 hours per month: 425.8 hours per month in St Omer, 417.9 hours per month in La Manche, and 247.1 hours per month in Athis Mons.

• For all three areas, and at both the second and third assessments, there was a clear correlation between the probability of receipt of informal care and the user's level of dependency.

Formal service response

• By the time of the second assessment, 81.5 per cent of users in St Omer were receiving formal help with household tasks, compared with 50.0 per cent in Athis Mons and 41.2 per cent in La Manche. Although the proportion varied, the ranking remained the same at the time of the third assessment: 76.5 per cent, 60.0 per cent and 51.4 per cent respectively.

• Formal help for personal care tasks, however, showed a more even pattern at the time of the second assessment, it being received by 50.0 per cent of users in Athis Mons, 48.1 per cent in St Omer and 41.2 per cent in La Manche.

• By the third assessment, the ranking had changed, with 43.2 per cent of users receiving formal help for personal care tasks in La Manche, 42 per cent in Athis Mons and 35.8 per cent in St Omer.

• The average number of hours of formal help received by users for any tasks at the time of the second assessment was 53.6 hours per month: 54.6 hours per month in Athis Mons, 69.5 hours per month in La Manche, and 35.6 hours per month in St Omer.

• For users receiving services for any tasks at the time of the third assessment, the ranking between areas remained the same, but the number of hours per month which users received had changed to 53.1

3 Fieldworkers at the French site were asked to specify who performed what task for the user at what time of day and on which day(s) of the week. The difficulty of estimating how much time an informal carer spends on tasks such as shopping which could be for the benefit of someone other than exclusively for the user, while possibly reduced by this approach, still means that these figures should be treated with some reserve.

hours per month in Athis Mons, 110.1 hours per month in La Manche, and 27.2 hours per month in St Omer.

- For 46.5 per cent of users in all three sites who by the time of the second assessment, were receiving the cash allowance ACTP there was a relative who was not a spouse who was an informal caregiver.

Destinational outcomes for users

- By the time of the second assessment, the highest proportion of users remaining at home was in St Omer: 61.4 per cent compared with 56.0 per cent in Athis Mons and 54.2 per cent in La Manche.
- By the time of the third assessment, however, the highest proportion of users remaining at home was in La Manche, at 80.8 per cent of those users who had been at home at the time of the second assessment, compared with 72.5 per cent for Athis Mons and 63.0 per cent for St Omer.
- Of those users who had left home by the time of the second assessment, the principal cause in St Omer was through entry into residential care, 11.5 per cent. For users in La Manche and Athis Mons, the principal cause was death: 23.0 per cent and 24.6 per cent respectively.
- At the time of the third assessment, while death remained the main cause in La Manche, at 13.5 per cent, users in Athis Mons and St Omer were most likely to cease to receive home care services because of entry into some form of institutional care: 8.4 per cent and 18.1 per cent respectively.

2. Key features

2.1. Contrasting foci: direct influence on supply versus subsidisation with regulation

Chapter 2 described how the historic emphasis of English policy has been the creation and operation of an efficient supply system. England has only recently awoken to the fact that policy has not hitherto been developed to help in the creation of suitable mechanisms for the private financing of dependency care for an elderly population of which the majority of members are neither poor enough to be eligible for state benefits, nor affluent enough to be able to pay for long-term care without serious if not catastrophic consequences for non-dependent spouses. The issue was raised by academics during the mid-eighties. Sir Roy Griffiths' report recognised its importance. However, it was not treated as a priority in the reform of community care during the late eighties. It was only in the early eighties that the discussion acquired sufficient political momentum for the creation of an interdepartmental committee focused on it. During 1996 and 1997, there were two white papers proposing a framework for partnership schemes based on the ideas of the Connecticut Partnership, now the basis of development in some American states. The Institute for Public Policy Research sponsored a report from London Economics proposing a Partial Equity Release Insurance scheme (PERI) (Richards, 1996). The Joseph Rowntree Foundation Inquiry (1996) recommended a National Care Insurance scheme, compulsory social insurance to cover care costs (without means-testing) and accommodation costs (subject to means-tested copayment if the benefits are insufficient to cover costs). The Labour Party is to establish a Royal Commission. There is also a Millennium Commission inquiry into alternative funding scenarios.

In contrast, as we described in Chapter 3, the French have always used financing mechanisms as a main instrument for achieving policy goals. Whereas at the end of the Second World War the English established a state-dominated system for the supply and coordination of community care for the majority of the population, the French built on the multiplicity of existing institutions.

This has caused the definition of policy issues to be different. However, French policy-making opinion also looked at the policy for the financing of long-term care with new eyes from the late nineties. The opening section alluded to a ferment of debate, followed by policy experimentation: the proposals for a new *prestation dépendance* in the Boulard (Assemblé nationale, 1991) and Schopflin reports (Commissariat général du plan, 1991); the aborted proposals of the Bérégovoy administration; the commitments made in the presidential election campaign of 1994; and the *prestation autonomie* whose implementation was postponed in November 1995, which was considered in the French parliament at the end of 1996, was promised from the beginning of 1997, partially tested in the twelve demonstration projects with forms of the *prestation experimentale dépendance* but finally replaced by the more modest *prestation spécifique dépendance*.

2.2. *Implications of the contrast*

What our research contributes to the debate follows from some of the facts discovered.

Mixed social insurance and social assistance financing
We have pointed to the contrast between the La Manche collections and the other French sites.The significance is the different weight of the collection towards financing from the *aide sociale* provided by the *département* in La Manche.

The summary shows substantial differences. The accounts of the workings of the systems in other ways illustrates one case of arrangements which mix social insurance and social assistance financing. It is a case in which the social insurance financing is based on variable but, in comparison for instance with the Israeli long-term care insurance, relatively generous qualifying criteria for benefit. The Joseph Rowntree Foundation appeared to be proposing a mixed system, since the report made no mention of denying to social services departments the right to use local authority revenue to subsidise services for persons not qualifying by the standard national criteria. Should a British mixed system combine more generous qualifying criteria for social insurance with more stringent criteria for social assistance benefits, there could be differences like those between the La Manche patterns and the others. However, it is more likely that the qualifying criteria for social insurance would be stringent, so that it could be made into an entitlement claimable by the beneficiary on the basis of agreed criteria, without massive leakage of funding to those who could find alternative means of support without great disbenefits in the absence of benefit. In that case, the local authority criteria might be more generous and more discretionary. The pattern then would be more like the mixing of direct state and more stringent third-party Medicaid funding in the USA, save that Medicaid there is a social assistance programme (Kassner and Williams, 1997).

Targeting cash with brokerage
The French *allocation compensatrice*, roughly the equivalent of English attendance allowances, is targeted, and varies more between users. Those receiving it can have access to brokerage help. Chapter 6 attempts to compare its marginal productivity with English benefits and inputs

of services in kind. Our results show that variations in *allocation compensatrice* have much greater apparent effects on the probabilities of admission to institutions for long-term care than the British equivalent. That is so, though both systems have been alleged to have some of the same vices and virtues.

The importance to French argument is that the results suggest that, whatever happens to the *prestation dépendance* in the period of fiscal adjustment during the next few years, policy should build on the strength of a targeted, broker-assisted benefit.

The importance for English policy analysts is that it puts into question whether such cash benefits intended to compensate for the costs of coping with declining independence in the performance of the tasks of daily living as attendance allowances should be treated separately from the system of subsidised community care services in kind. The marginal productivities of the expenditures on each should be compared. Each should be made to complement the other. It could just be that the productivity of the English attendance allowance has been improved by the attempts of local authorities to purloin it for the payment of their charges to users. But the uncoordinated and varying policy initiatives of local authorities can hardly be expected to produce a coherent and consistent improvement in equity, broadly defined.

Marginal productivities of services

The English community social services in kind have a higher average productivity given their levels of input and targeting than their French counterparts, an effect which is much greater than the difference in the supply of places in homes. New recipients of community-based services in France had twice the probability of admission to institutions for long-term care than a matched sample of new recipients in England. The descriptions in Chapter 3 may provide some of the explanations: the more fragmented system in France, financial incentives, the implied judgement that the flows of finance are not so subsidised from state funds that arrangements should ensure the best use of public funds in providing incentives to users to choose one mode rather than another. Another reason why the issue has not been formulated in the same way in France is because French research has focused not on variations in individual costs of care irrespective of mode, but on averages for levels of dependency and the like.

The implication is that the French should consider accelerating their attempts to secure coordination of commissioning for individuals, and the consolidation of provision by supply agencies. The arrangements for the *prestation spécifique dépendance* may provide sharp incentives to national and local financing and providing agencies. But the incentives lack finesse. The French have relied on voluntary cooperation at the local level in a wide range of social policy areas (Evans et al., 1995). Our areas included some which were among the more coordinated of French systems. But, as argued by the Schopflin report and others, resources are not matched to need. Reflecting the absence of authority and legitimacy for any one agency to force through change against the opposition and reluctance of vested interests, the French approach to agency coordination at the local level is reminiscent of attempts in the fragmented American system, for instance the Long-Term Care Planning Council of the State of New York during the eighties, rather than the development of trade and industry policies in the best British authorities.

The English development of case management could be of value in France, as evidence about its working and effects in practice in the nationwide routine implementation becomes available to supplement the experiments conducted during the last decade (Davies et al., 1990; Davies, 1992). Again, the English might have useful experience in the management of the development of local markets to create a mixed economy of care.

The marginal productivity of the English services in kind might be superior. Some evidence suggests that they have already been further improved by the reforms. There is evidence of lower use of residential care due to more intensive and need-matched home care, and of increases in the length of stay in the community associated with each level of input (Davies et al., 1995b, 1996a,b,c). These are some of the main improvements sought from the contemporary reforms.

But the post-reform gains in England and Wales too are smaller than could be achieved. Chapter 2 illustrates the way in which British local authorities only partially implemented some of the principles of budget-devolved care management. Accessible literature remains unread, illustrating a Department of Health comment that social services remains an 'oral culture'. Authorities have excessively leant on advice from the Department of Health. Such a medium could not have been expected to have taught logical principle, technological knowledge of the variety of kinds needed by persons performing several different functions, and an analytic approach to the creation of care management arrangements, with as much success as university departments taught such things to town planners.

Whether and how quickly the improvements are achieved will be of interest to other countries. To put it crudely, have the improvements been fast enough to make the supply-side reform of care systems worth the political effort?

The displacement of informal care by services

The collection of data for France allowed a more thorough analysis of the degree to which the provision of services by agencies displaced care from relatives and other 'informal sources' than has hitherto been avail- able in the international literature. The advance was made possible by the collection of the opinions about the number of hours from each source given to each task for each case, and the creation of a range of new indicators of aspects of displacement and related phenomena.

The most important questions are not for what proportion of users is the care from informal sources displaced by care from agencies, and in cases of such displacement how great is the displacement. The important questions are for what proportion of users is there is a displacement which cannot be justified by the situation of the user or informal care-givers, and how great is the unjustifiable displacement.

Chapter 6 investigates the proportion of cases for which unjustifiable displacement is probable. Attempts to take into account complicating factors reduced the numbers and the extent of the substitution. It concluded that unjustifiable displacement was likely for only a low proportion of cases, probably less than 8 per cent of cases. However, for some among those for which the displacement might have been unjustified, the amount of displacement was large. Like the measurement of marginal productivities, the estimation of unjustifiable displacement is necessarily subject to a large margin of error. However, as in the comparison of the marginal productivities, the general conclusion is relatively clear. In this, the results for France are similar to results using cruder indicators for the UK and USA (Tennstedt et al., 1993).

The implication for France is that the system has enough checks and balances to prevent a degree of unjustifiable displacement. In particular, France has the Napoleonic *obligation alimentaire*. No doubt, some of the vices alleged by the Schopflin report and other critiques contribute to the apparently low degree of displacement: the failure to provide what is most needed and wanted, among them contributions to alleviating needs catered for by informal caregivers.

The dangers are more likely to arise in systems which combine two features: narrow limits to the responsibilities of partners and relatives for caring; and the provision of attractive and effective forms of community services closely matching the needs and wishes of users and informal caregivers. That is the intent of the British community care reforms. In effect, the full implementation of their rhetoric would for many users remove some of the most important deterrent effects of the workhouse test and the principle of less eligibility: the loss of autonomy, the freedom to exercise authority and choice over one's day-to-day life, and the acceptance of services which are demeaning. There are countervailing factors: the requirement for copayment and the increasing pressure of need-generated demand on public subsidies. Therefore, it will be interesting to examine substitution in the post-reform history of English authorities which are on the one hand doing most to implement high-quality community services in ways which reflect needs and wishes, and which on the other hand have more adequate growth in their service budgets. However, the results of such analyses are not yet available.

3. Current reforms: sound foundations for the future?

We must think also of the longer run.

3.1. England and Wales

In the UK, the new policy structures and processes have unleashed a new dynamic which will power change for many years to come. Indeed, there seems to have been a conscious choice in community care as in health policy to give precedence to making radical structural change, and so to unleash fundamentally new processes. The logic was *perestroika* and *glasnost*: a retreat from a supply-led system based on fitting persons to the narrow range of standard services planned into the future with Soviet hubris with data of almost Soviet inaccuracy. It was to create structures which would create incentives to improve outcomes, to create a plurality of suppliers whose competition in response to the incentives would lead to improved efficiency and development of new ways of achieving goals, to create managed markets as the vehicle for this incentive-led change, to empower consumers at least to some extent, and to a greater extent increase their direct and indirect influence mediated through the new case management brokers and others.

Many managers and providers have believed in, and have acted out, the traditional Anglo-Saxon concept of the competitive process of the kind taught in the most elementary textbooks. Middle managers in the social services departments are in many authorities vigorously seeking the lowest prices for residential care compatible with acceptable quality. Suppliers who fail to compete effectively are leaving the market. The dangers of price competition with an excessive concern of the purchasers in the short run compared with the long run are very real. These beliefs, and the behaviours which they are encouraging, are thus enhancing the risks of the market failures which much of that literature has explored.

It is true that Ministers no longer use the words competition and the market. They stress cooperative long-run relationships between the community care authorities who purchase, provide quality assurance, and in other ways develop and implement 'trade and industry' policies. To a great extent, this simply reflects the shift from the naive view that the policy-makers had of the nature of the competitive process; that what is now being stressed is more a competitive process of the type discussed by the Austrian School than of Anglo-Saxon economists of the thirties and before. It is only now that academics are producing reviews of the academic economic theory of most relevance to the new community care context; for instance Forder et al. (1996).

However, it is unlikely that the increased sophistication as time passes will replace the price/quality competition now established. It is more likely that managers will resort to the usual repertoire of trade and industry policies to attempt to remove structural imperfections of the markets leading to market failures: attempt to overcome obstacles to entry, thus making markets more 'contestable' in the long run if the present suppliers fail to satisfy; maintaining competitiveness by blocking mergers and the like; using such techniques as 'franchising' to overcome such barriers to exit as high sunk costs; sometimes setting floors or ceilings to prices as well as quality; and tuning the combinations of these partially incompatible means to the context and the time — that is, behaving with that broad repertoire of trade and industry policy which is seen in many other areas of the economy.

With this emphasis on the structures and ideologies which influence action, it is a contradiction also to try to specify the precise nature of what should be supplied. However, one can describe some of the mismatches which restrict the capacity of the new system to deliver. One obvious mismatch is between what home care provides, and what is needed by different groups of users. The starting point should be the need-related circumstances of disabled elderly people and caregivers. A typology based on these circumstances through time would suggest quite different content and organisation of provision, both of the home care services and of 'shelter-with-care'. It is from the imaginative definition of such typologies, and from matching their elements to some of the exciting models being developed but as yet only at a small scale throughout the francophone and Anglo-Saxon worlds — such models as the *cantou* and On Lok — that there will be the analytic frameworks to help the new arrangements to work. What this amounts to is the promotion of service vision by juxtaposing insights about the effects of flows of provision, about needs, and about market demand. The argument is developed elsewhere (Davies, 1998).

The British case is extreme. In no other major country has there been this same reconstruction from first principles. However, there are other major countries pursuing some of the same goals, with slightly different emphases.

3.2. *France*

As distant observers of French care policy, we think that we can see a danger that France may not join this group of pioneers in the adventure of reconstructing community and long-term care from its foundations. The institutions make change difficult. The corporatism which has contributed in so many other ways to the success of France during a quarter of a century or more may prevent such radical reconstruction. The timing of the reform movement has been unlucky. It is a few years too late. Other national goals may take precedence in the short run, and continue to demand the subjugation of other policy goals in the long run, like the consolidation of the Union by establishing the common currency.

Yet there may be a confluence of several streams during the next few years. The new allowance, the PSD, was introduced as an interim provision during the final days of the last right-wing government under Prime Minister Juppé. The new socialist government has not expressed any firm views on the operation of the allowance, despite repeated calls on the health minister, Mme Martine Aubry, to review its operation both at the level of the operation of the actual allowance or, more profoundly, by relocating responsibility for it from the local authorities to the state social security system.[4] By this means, the new government retains its freedom of action to undertake any reforms which may become necessary as local authorities increasingly struggle to finance both the actual allowance and its management, and with the requirement for more fieldwork staff to undertake even the minimum care management role required by the legislation.[5]

The location of responsibility for the PSD with the *départements* rather than with the *Sécu* and the *Caisse nationale d'assurance maladie* (CNAM) was probably a result of political pressures, with the former government needing the support of the Sénat, whose members, thanks the French habit of *cumul des mandats*, were often also important members of the local *conseils généraux*, and so keen to secure control of the new allowance from CNAM. Equally, central government, seeking to control its own expenditure in order to qualify for entry to European Monetary Union (EMU), saw advantage in passing responsibility for what would no doubt prove to be an expensive allowance to local authorities.

Over the next few years, as EMU moves towards implementation, another of Jospin's legislative programmes, that to limit the *cumul des mandats*, may be starting to have effect. At the same time, both local authorities in the operation of the PSD, and CNAM with its continued

4 See Chapter 3.

5 The *Dernières Nouvelles d'Alsace* of 23 February 1998 reports that, over the first year of operation of the PSD, 534 whole-time equivalent employees had been recruited by the *conseils généraux*.

provision of domiciliary care, will have gained experience in forms of care-managed home care. By then, the tensions for the local authorities in implementing the PSD not integrated with the social action provision of *assurance maladie* might have become clear to even the most forthright defender of the primacy of the *conseils généraux*, the members of which may have also lost some wider political influence at the national level. So it is possible that there may be a reform of the PSD by the socialist government, perhaps on the lines of the integrated financing of domiciliary care first seen in the experimental projects such as that in the Ille et Vilaine. The current reforms to the financing of the health care budget, with its moves towards a generalised tax-based model through the *contribution sociale généralisée* (CSG), rather than continuing with the insurance model of employment-related contributions, is yet another, although at this stage separate, indicator of the fundamental direction of change within the French welfare model.

This would leave untouched another main strand of community care logic: creating incentives to choose between home care and various forms of shelter-with-care which reflect a coherent set of judgements about what would improve equity and efficiency at the level of the individual and the family. But again, we have yet to see the application of the new PSD to residents in both social and health financed care beds, and the reform of the tariffication of such beds so that funding is related not to the category of each bed but rather the dependency level of its occupant. This could well lead to closer rather than weaker links between the funding of the two forms of care provision. This, however, is speculative; other close observers of the French scene for care of older people are less optimistic. Starting from the premise that, for the French government, care of the elderly is a much lower priority than dealing with unemployment and controlling the overall social security bill, they would argue that the present interim PSD will not be radically reformed but rather left to wither into a form of minimal allowance for the least well-off elderly, with all others being left no alternative but to seek some form of private insurance.

Either scenario would clearly lead to a radically different model of social care for France than that examined here, and will certainly make it worthwhile to undertake another study of the same kind in a decade's time.

Annex: Need-related circumstances, caregiver and service responses and destinational outcomes during two years: the French sites compared

A.1. Introduction

The present section provides basic descriptives for the French sample for the second and third assessments. First, it focuses on destinational data: specifically on the pattern of attrition, crude outcomes for people leaving the community, and the comparison of dependency measures (the French functional INSERM categories and the English Isaacs and Neville, 1975, disability levels) by outcomes. Then it describes the levels of informal and formal care, and the informal care response to levels of dependency by specific tasks, initially and through time.

A.2. Destinational tables: proportions remaining in the community after the second and third assessments

Tables A.1 and A.2 show a deceleration in the rate of attrition between two periods: between the first and second assessments, and between the second and third assessments. This could be due to high numbers of cases leaving the community soon after first assessment not being able to cope with the 'crisis' that brought them into the system. Since in the main the fitter would remain after this first phase, the proportions of cases leaving the community at the time of subsequent assessments would be lower.

The proportions of cases remaining in the community vary between areas at second and third assessments. At the second assessment, higher proportions remained in the community in St Omer compared with La Manche and Athis Mons (61 per cent against 56 and 54 per cent

Table A.1. Whether client still in community at time two: proportions of persons by area

		Yes	Total
Athis Mons	row %	54.2	100.0
	no.	32	59
La Manche	row %	56.0	100.0
	no.	51	91
St Omer	row %	61.4	100.0
	no.	27	44
Total	%	56.7	100.0
	no.	110	194

Tests of significance:

Difference between all 3 areas: p=.759, applying a Chi-square test.
Difference between each area and other areas individually:
Between Athis Mons and La Manche: p=.829, applying a t-test.
Between Athis Mons and St Omer: p=.474, applying a t-test.
Between La Manche and St Omer: p=.561, applying a t-test.

Table A.2. Whether client still in community at time three: proportions of persons by area

		Yes	Total
Athis Mons	row %	80.8	100.0
	no.	21	26
La Manche	row %	72.5	100.0
	no.	29	40
St Omer	row %	63.0	100.0
	no.	17	27
Total	%	72.0	100.0
	no.	67	93

Tests of significance:

Difference between all 3 areas: p=.351, applying a Chi-square test.
Between Athis Mons and La Manche: p=.451, applying a t-test.
Between Athis Mons and St Omer: p=.156, applying a t-test.
Between La Manche and St Omer: p=.417, applying a t-test.

Table A.3. Destination of client at time two: proportions of persons by area

		INSERM category				With-drew	Total
		grp 4	grp 3	grp 2	grp 1		
Athis Mons	row %	8.8	15.8	31.6	.0	5.3	100.0
	no.	5	9	18	0	3	57
La Manche	row %	3.4	5.7	43.7	5.7	.0	100.0
	no.	3	5	38	5	0	87
St Omer	row %	9.1	20.5	31.8	.0	6.8	100.0
	no.	4	9	14	0	3	44
Total	row %	6.4	12.2	37.2	2.7	3.2	100.0
	no.	12	23	70	5	6	188
		Moved	*Long-stay*	*Res. home*	*Foster home*	*Died*	*Total*
Athis Mons	row %	3.5	5.3	5.3	.0	24.6	100.0
	no.	2	3	3	0	14	57
La Manche	row %	1.1	1.1	16.1	.0	23.0	100.0
	no.	1	1	14	0	20	87
St Omer	row %	4.5	11.4	4.5	2.3	9.1	100.0
	no.	2	5	2	1	4	44
Total	row %	2.7	4.8	10.1	.5	20.2	100.0
	no.	5	9	19	1	38	188

Tests of significance:

Difference between all 3 areas: p=.001, applying a Chi-square test.
Difference between each area and other areas individually:
Between Athis Mons and La Manche: p=.844, applying a t-test.
Between Athis Mons and St Omer: p=.385, applying a t-test.
Between La Manche and St Omer: p=.257, applying a t-test.

Table A.4. Destination of client at time three: proportions of persons by area

		Grp 4	Grp 3	Grp 2	Grp 1	Client moved	Total
Athis Mons	row %	20.8	37.5	29.2			100.0
	col %	38.5	64.3	19.4			
	no.	5	9	7			24
La Manche	row %	8.1		64.9	5.4	5.4	100.0
	col %	23.1		66.7	50.0	100.0	
	no.	3		24	2	2	37
St Omer	row %	22.7	22.7	22.7	9.1		100.0
	col %	38.5	35.7	13.9	50.0		
	no.	5	5	5	2		22
Total	row %	15.7	16.9	43.4	4.8	5.4	100.0
	col %	100.0	100.0	100.0	100.0	100.0	100.0
	no.	13	14	36	4	2	83

Destination of client at time three (continued)

		Long-stay	Res. home	Foster home	Died	Total
Athis Mons	row %	4.2	4.2		4.2	100.0
	col %	25.0	50.0		14.3	
	no.	1	1		1	24
La Manche	row %		2.7		13.5	100.0
	col %		50.0		71.4	
	no.		1		5	37
St Omer	row %	13.6		4.5	4.5	100.0
	col %	75.0		100.0	14.3	
	no.	3		1	1	22
Total	row %	4.8	2.4	1.2	8.4	100.0
	col %	100.0	100.0	100.0	100.0	100.0
	no.	4	2	1	7	83

respectively). The reverse is true at third assessment. In St Omer 63 per cent of the cases remained in community compared with 73 per cent in La Manche and 81 per cent in Athis Mons.

A.3. Destination of the French sample by INSERM categories of disability

Table A.5 shows the French sample's destination by their INSERM category. INSERM groups 2, 3 and 4 show great stability, with 60 per cent, 40 per cent and 53 per cent of the cases respectively remaining within their original category (destination at second assessment). On the contrary, cases in INSERM group 1 at first assessment are scattered across different outcomes at second assessment. Only 8 per cent of the cases originally labelled group 1 remained in group 1 at second assessment.

INSERM categorisation does not appear to be a good predictor of either entry into shelter-with-care or morbidity. Indeed, less than half of the cases entering residential care by the second assessment came from INSERM group 1, the highest disability INSERM category. Only one-third of those cases who died were from that group.

The equivalent table for destination at time three, Table A.6, shows a similar pattern, though the small numbers prevent further analysis.

A.4. Destinations of French sample relative to the original level of disability measured by interval need

When the measure of dependency used is interval need, the Isaacs and Neville scale, much higher proportions of cases are placed in the category for the highest level of dependency than when the INSERM scale is used as the measure for dependency (34.6 per cent for the INSERM categorisation compared with 62.2 per cent for Isaacs and Neville at first assessment).

Perhaps this is not surprising because the sample is of cases presenting for some form of social care, and the Isaacs and Neville scale is a measure of need for interventions rather than a more absolute measure of task performance. Certainly the Isaacs and Neville categorisation seems to be a good predictor of outcomes, since Tables A.7 and A.8 suggest the evolution of dependency be primarily deterioration rather than the more mixed pattern presented in the tables using the INSERM categorisation. For the most dependent cases tables based on the Isaacs

Table A.5. Destination of client at time two and INSERM category at first assessment: proportions of persons overall

		INSERM category at first assessment				
		Grp 4	*Grp 3*	*Grp 2*	*Grp 1*	*Total*
Client's destination at time two						
Group 4	row %	100.0				100.0
	col %	60.0				
	no.	12				12
Group 3	row %	8.7	78.3	4.3	8.7	100.0
	col %	10.0	40.0	1.7	3.1	
	no.	2	18	1	2	23
Group 2	row %	1.4	18.6	44.3	35.7	100.0
	col %	5.0	28.9	53.4	38.5	
	no.	1	13	31	25	70
Group 1	row %				100.0	100.0
	col %				7.7	
	no.				5	5
Client withdrew	row %	16.7	16.7	66.7		100.0
	col %	5.0	2.2	6.9		
	no.	1	1	4		6
Client moved	row %		40.0	20.0	40.0	100.0
	col %		4.4	1.7	3.1	
	no.		2	1	2	5
Permanent place long-stay	row %			55.6	44.4	100.0
	col %			8.6	6.2	
	no.			5	4	9
Permanent place residential	row %	15.8	10.5	31.6	42.1	100.0
	col %	15.0	4.4	10.3	12.3	
	no.	3	2	6	8	19
Permanent place foster home	row %		100.0			100.0
	col %		2.2			
	no.		1			1
Client died	row %	2.6	21.1	26.3	50.0	100.0
	col %	5.0	17.8	17.2	29.2	
	no.	1	8	10	19	38
Total	row %	10.6	23.9	30.9	34.6	100.0
	col %	100.0	100.0	100.0	100.0	100.0
	no.	20	45	58	65	

Table A.6. Destination of client at time three and INSERM category at time two: proportions of persons overall

		INSERM category at time two				
		Grp 4	Grp 3	Grp 2	Grp 1	Total
Client's destination at time three						
Group 4	row %	84.6	15.4			100.0
	col %	91.7	9.5			
	no.	11	2			13
Group 3	row %		85.7	14.3		100.0
	col %		57.1	4.3		
	no.		12	2		14
Group 2	row %		8.3	91.7		100.0
	col %		14.3	71.7		
	no.		3	33		36
Group 1	row %		25.0	25.0	50.0	100.0
	col %		4.8	2.2	50.0	
	no.		1	1	2	4
Moved	row %			100.0		100.0
	col %			4.3		
	no.			2		2
Permanent place long-stay	row %		50.0	50.0		100.0
	col %		9.5	4.3		
	no.		2	2		4
Permanent place residential	row %					100.0
	col %					
	no.					2
Permanent place foster home	row %		100.0			100.0
	col %		4.8			
	no.		1			1
Client died	row %	14.3		57.1	28.6	100.0
	col %	8.3		8.7	50.0	
	no.	1		4	2	7
Total	row %	14.5	25.3	55.4	4.8	100.0
	col %	100.0	100.0	100.0	100.0	100.0
	no.	12	21	46	4	83

Table A.7. Destination of client at time two and interval need level at first assessment: proportions of persons overall

		Interval need level at first assessment				
		Ind.	*Long*	*Short*	*Crit.*	*Total*
Client's destination at time two						
Independent	row %	75.0			25.0	100.0
	col %	75.0			1.7	
	no.	6			2	8
Long	row %	11.1	66.7	22.2		100.0
	col %	12.5	42.9	4.1		
	no.	1	6	2		9
Short	row %	3.7	7.4	63.0	25.9	100.0
	col %	12.5	14.3	34.7	6.0	
	no.	1	2	17	7	27
Critical	row %		1.5	15.2	83.3	100.0
	col %		7.1	20.4	47.0	
	no.		1	10	55	66
Client withdrew	row %		16.7	66.7	16.7	100.0
	col %		7.1	8.2	.9	
	no.		1	4	1	6
Client moved	row %				100.0	100.0
	col %				4.3	
	no.				5	5
Permanent place long-stay	row %			44.4	55.6	100.0
	col %			8.2	4.3	
	no.			4	5	9
Permanent place residential	row %			31.6	68.4	100.0
	col %			12.2	11.1	
	no.			6	13	19
Permanent place foster home	row %				100.0	100.0
	col %				.9	
	no.				1	1
Client died	row %		10.5	15.8	73.7	100.0
	col %		28.6	12.2	23.9	
	no.		4	6	28	38
Total	row %	4.3	7.4	26.1	62.2	100.0
	col %	100.0	100.0	100.0	100.0	100.0
	no.	8	14	49	117	188

Table A.8. Destination of client at time three and interval need level at time two: proportions of persons overall

		Interval need level at time two				
		Ind.	*Long*	*Short*	*Crit.*	*Total*
Client's destination at time three						
Independent	row %	66.7	11.1	11.1	11.1	100.0
	col %	66.7	11.1	4.2	1.7	
	no.	6	1	1	1	9
Long	row %	8.3	41.7	8.3	41.7	100.0
	col %	11.1	55.6	4.2	8.6	
	no.	1	5	1	5	12
Short	row %		6.7	86.7	6.7	100.0
	col %		11.1	54.2	1.7	
	no.		1	13	1	15
Critical	row %	4.7		11.6	83.7	100.0
	col %	22.2		20.8	62.1	
	no.	2		5	36	43
Client moved	row %			33.3	66.7	100.0
	col %			4.2	3.4	
	no.			1	2	3
Permanent place long-stay	row %		25.0	25.0	50.0	100.0
	col %		11.1	4.2	3.4	
	no.		1	1	2	4
Permanent place residential	row %		33.3		66.7	100.0
	col %		11.1		3.4	
	no.		1		2	3
Permanent place foster care	row %				100.0	100.0
	col %				1.7	
	no.				1	1
Client died	row %			20.0	80.0	100.0
	col %			8.3	13.8	
	no.			2	8	10
Total	row %	9.0	9.0	24.0	58.0	100.0
	col %	100.0	100.0	100.0	100.0	100.0
	no.	9	9	24	58	100

and Neville categorisation, the change through time again corresponds well to the pattern that could be expected, with cases tending to either remain at home but be very dependent, with no significant improvement in functioning, or entering some form of institutional care, or dying. This suggests that the Isaacs and Neville measures of dependency are better predictors of outcomes in the field of social care, certainly when compared with the more medically oriented measure that is the basis of the INSERM categorisation, since it is based upon the degree of need for external intervention to assist with any particular task. The Isaacs and Neville categorisation therefore reflects more accurately the demands the particular individual will make upon those in a position to help. The INSERM categorisation, however, being more focused on the ability of an individual to perform specific tasks, regardless of the social circumstances, reflects a more insurance-based model of welfare founded on individual entitlements.

A.5. Informal response to needs

Looked at across time, as in Tables A.9 and A.10, the proportions of cases getting informal help tend to diminish. La Manche consistently remains the area where the highest proportions of cases receive such help, followed first by Athis Mons and then St Omer, which in addition shows substantially lower proportions of the samples with recorded inputs of informal help. This may be due to the small number of married cases in St Omer, and to the presence of the cash benefit of ACTP in La Manche, which would encourage the 'payment' of informal helpers, and therefore increase the probability of getting informal help.

By the time of the second assessment there is a clear positive correlation between the presence of informal help and levels of disability. This is so for all three areas. The pattern is not as clear for the third assessment, particularly for Athis Mons, where cases receiving informal help in the highest dependency category fall from 89 per cent at the second assessment to 64 per cent at the time of the third. The small number overall of cases by the time of the third assessment, however, undermines the statistical significance of the proportions shown in Table A.10.

Table A.9. INSERM need category and presence of informal help with any task at time two: proportions of persons by area

		Yes	*Total*
Athis Mons			
Group 4	row %	80.0	100.0
	col %	15.4	
	no.	4	5
Group 3	row %	66.7	100.0
	col %	23.1	
	no.	6	9
Group 2	row %	88.9	100.0
	col %	61.5	
	no.	16	18
Total	row %	81.3	100.0
	col %	100.0	
	no.	26	32
La Manche			
Group 4	row %	100.0	100.0
	col %	6.1	
	no.	3	3
Group 3	row %	100.0	100.0
	col %	10.2	
	no.	5	5
Group 2	row %	94.7	100.0
	col %	73.5	
	no.	36	38
Group 1	row %	100.0	100.0
	col %	10.2	
	no.	5	5
Total	row %	96.1	100.0
	col %	100.0	
	no.	49	51
St Omer			
Group 4	row %		100.0
	col %		
	no.		4
Group 3	row %		100.0
	col %		
	no.		9
Group 2	row %	71.4	100.0
	col %	100.0	
	no.	10	14
Total	row %	37.0	100.0
	col %	100.0	
	no.	10	27

Table A.10. INSERM need category and presence of informal help with any task at time three: proportions of persons by area

		Yes	Total
Athis Mons			
Group 4	row %	80.0	100.0
	col %	22.0	
	no.	4	5
Group 3	row %	77.8	100.0
	col %	38.9	
	no.	7	9
Group 2	row %	63.6	100.0
	col %	38.9	
	no.	7	11
Total	row %	72.0	100.0
	col %	100.0	
	no.	18	25
La Manche			
Group 4	row %	75.0	100.0
	col %	8.8	
	no.	3	4
Group 2	row %	93.1	100.0
	col %	79.4	
	no.	27	29
Group 1	row %	100.0	100.0
	col %	11.8	
	no.	4	4
Total	row %	91.9	100.0
	col %	100.0	
	no.	34	37
St Omer			
Group 4	row %		100.0
	col %		
	no.		5
Group 3	row %		100.0
	col %		
	no.		5
Group 2	row %	60.0	100.0
	col %	60.0	
	no.	3	5
Group 1	row %	100.0	100.0
	col %	40.0	
	no.	2	2
Total	row %	29.4	100.0
	col %	100.0	
	no.	5	17

Table A.11. Presence of informal help with personal care at time two: proportions of persons by area

		Yes	*Total*
Athis Mons	row %	28.1	100.0
	no.	9	32
La Manche	row %	76.6	100.0
	no.	36	51
St Omer	row %	18.5	100.0
	no.	5	27
Total	%	45.5	100.0
	no.	50	110

Tests of significance:
Difference between all 3 areas: p=.000, applying a Chi-square test.
Difference between each area and other areas individually:
Between Athis Mons and La Manche: p=.000, applying a t-test.
Between Athis Mons and St Omer: p=.390, applying a t-test.
Between La Manche and St Omer: p=.000, applying a t-test.

A.6. Informal care in relation to specific tasks

Tables A.11 to A.18 describe the contribution of informal care to specific tasks, such as personal care, household tasks and nutrition, where these are required. The ranking between areas is shown. There is no change in the pattern either for type of task or between assessments, with La Manche being the area where there is the highest level of informal help, followed by Athis Mons and then St Omer. There is some observable reduction in the informal inputs, however, between the second and third assessments, as was noted earlier.

A.7. Mean number of hours of informal help

As the previous tables have shown, there is a reduction across time in the numbers of cases which receive informal help inputs. When the mean of hours per month of this informal help is taken, however, there is a more mixed pattern, with some tasks, such as help with personal care or nutrition, showing an increase at the time of the third assessment compared with that at the time of the second. This could be expected

Table A.12. Presence of informal help with personal care at time three: proportions of persons by area

		Yes	Total
Athis Mons	row %	24.0	100.0
	no.	6	25
La Manche	row %	56.8	100.0
	no.	21	37
St Omer	row %	17.6	100.0
	no.	3	17
Total	%	38.0	100.0
	no.	30	79

Tests of significance:
Difference between all 3 areas: p=.0003, applying a Chi-square test.
Difference between each area and other areas individually:
Between Athis Mons and La Manche: p=.0082, applying a t-test.
Between Athis Mons and St Omer: p=.2701, applying a t-test.
Between La Manche and St Omer: p=.0062, applying a t-test.

Table A.13. Presence of informal help with household tasks at time two: proportions of persons by area

		Yes	Total
Athis Mons	row %	34.4	100.0
	no.	11	32
La Manche	row %	51.0	100.0
	no.	26	51
St Omer	row %	18.5	100.0
	no.	5	27
Total	%	38.2	100.0
	no.	42	110

Tests of significance:
Difference between all 3 areas: p=.017, applying a Chi-square test.
Difference between each area and other areas individually:
Between Athis Mons and La Manche: p=.139, applying a t-test.
Between Athis Mons and St Omer: p=.171, applying a t-test.
Between La Manche and St Omer: p=.003, applying a t-test.

Table A.14. Presence of informal help with household tasks at time three: proportions of persons by area

		Yes	*Total*
Athis Mons	row %	36.0	100.0
	no.	9	25
La Manche	row %	43.2	100.0
	no.	16	37
St Omer	row %	23.5	100.0
	no.	4	17
Total	%	36.7	100.0
	no.	29	79

Tests of significance:
Difference between all 3 areas: p=.0188, applying a Chi-square test.
Difference between each area and other areas individually:
Between Athis Mons and La Manche: p=.1785, applying a t-test.
Between Athis Mons and St Omer: p=.1905, applying a t-test.
Between La Manche and St Omer: p=.0954, applying a t-test.

Table A.15. Presence of informal help with nutrition at time two: proportions of persons by area

		Yes	*Total*
Athis Mons	row %	34.4	100.0
	no.	11	32
La Manche	row %	76.5	100.0
	no.	39	51
St Omer	row %	29.6	100.0
	no.	8	27
Total	%	52.7	100.0
	no.	58	110

Tests of significance:
Difference between all 3 areas: p=.000, applying a Chi-square test.
Difference between each area and other areas individually:
Between Athis Mons and La Manche: p=.000, applying a t-test.
Between Athis Mons and St Omer: p=.703, applying a t-test.
Between La Manche and St Omer: p=.000, applying a t-test.

Table A.16. Presence of informal help with nutrition at time three: proportions of persons by area

		Yes	*Total*
Athis Mons	row %	32.0	100.0
	no.	8	25
La Manche	row %	64.9	100.0
	no.	24	37
St Omer	row %	23.5	100.0
	no.	4	17
Total	%	45.6	100.0
	no.	36	79

Tests of significance:
Difference between all 3 areas: p=.0002, applying a Chi-square test.
Difference between each area and other areas individually:
Between Athis Mons and La Manche: p=.0085, applying a t-test.
Between Athis Mons and St Omer: p=.2328, applying a t-test.
Between La Manche and St Omer: p=.0045, applying a t-test.

Table A.17. Presence of informal help with shopping at time two: proportions of persons by area

		Yes	*Total*
Athis Mons	row %	68.8	100.0
	no.	22	32
La Manche	row %	84.3	100.0
	no.	43	51
St Omer	row %	33.3	100.0
	no.	9	27
Total	%	67.3	100.0
	no.	74	110

Tests of significance:
Difference between all 3 areas: p=.000, applying a Chi-square test.
Difference between each area and other areas individually:
Between Athis Mons and La Manche: p=.118, applying a t-test.
Between Athis Mons and St Omer: p=.006, applying a t-test.
Between La Manche and St Omer: p=.000, applying a t-test.

Table A.18. Presence of informal help with shopping at time three: proportions of persons by area

		Yes	*Total*
Athis Mons	row %	68.0	100.0
	no.	17	25
La Manche	row %	78.4	100.0
	no.	29	37
St Omer	row %	23.5	100.0
	no.	4	17
Total	%	63.3	100.0
	no.	50	79

Tests of significance:
Difference between all 3 areas: p=.0001, applying a Chi-square test.
Difference between each area and other areas individually:
Between Athis Mons and La Manche: p=.1528, applying a t-test.
Between Athis Mons and St Omer: p=.0096, applying a t-test.
Between La Manche and St Omer: p=.0002, applying a t-test.

Table A.19. Means of hours per month of informal help with any task by area at time two

	Mean	*Std dev*	*Cases*
For all areas	412.52	347.84	85
Athis Mons	296.13	401.17	26
La Manche	433.40	289.69	49
St Omer	612.83	383.86	10

Total cases = 85
Missing cases = 0
Test of signficance, p=.0387, applying analysis of variance

Table A.20. Means of hours per month of informal help with any task by area at time three

	Mean	*Std dev*	*Cases*
For all areas	364.65	369.02	57
Athis Mons	247.13	393.37	18
La Manche	417.87	363.52	34
St Omer	425.79	260.11	5

Total cases = 57
Missing cases = 0

in view of the pattern of increasing dependency of the recipients. St Omer ranks first, although it had the lowest actual number of cases receiving any informal care inputs. The small number of cases in many of the tasks does, though, make these estimated differences in mean numbers of hours per month of informal help of low statistical significance. The mean hours shown for the informal inputs for all tasks in Tables A.19 and A.20 must also be treated with caution, since the variable includes informal help providing companionship, an important component of domiciliary support but one which it is very difficult to quantify.

A.8. Formal response to needs

At the time of the second and third assessments, formal help is greater the higher is the level of dependency (Tables A.21 to A.30). This pattern was also noted in Chapter 6, Table 16, for the initial assessment. Over time, the proportions of cases receiving formal help remains constant. La Manche has consistently the lowest proportions of cases receiving formal help, reflecting no doubt the emphasis in that area on the use of the ACTP cash allowance.

At the time of the second assessment there are notable differences in the proportions of cases receiving help with household tasks, nutrition and shopping. St Omer has consistently higher proportions, followed by Athis Mons and finally La Manche. This pattern seems to remain through time, although the reduced number of cases at third assessment limits the reliability of the validity that the pattern observed in the sample is present in the population.

The pattern may be a reflection of the type of tasks undertaken by informal help (Tables A.11 to A.18). The findings reinforce the inference in Chapter 6 that the local formal care agencies seem to match their inputs to complement as far as possible the existing informal help.

The mean number of hours of formal help in the three areas shows over both the second and third periods of assessment higher levels of formal inputs allocated in La Manche. This is true for each type of task, however, but the proportions of cases in that area receiving formal help are smaller.

Table A.21. Means of hours per month of informal help with personal care by area at time two

	Mean	*Std dev*	*Cases*
For all areas	24.41	18.90	50
Athis Mons	16.85	15.84	9
La Manche	27.97	19.84	36
St Omer	12.37	2.95	5

Total cases = 50
Missing cases = 0
Test of signficance, p=.0915, applying analysis of variance

Table A.22. Means of hours per month of informal help with personal care by area at time three

	Mean	*Std dev*	*Cases*
For all areas	31.80	28.45	30
Athis Mons	13.28	8.29	6
La Manche	34.07	26.63	21
St Omer	53.00	52.16	3

Total cases = 30
Missing cases = 0

Table A.23. Means of hours per month of informal help with household tasks by area at time two

	Mean	*Std dev*	*Cases*
For all areas	31.17	21.76	42
Athis Mons	39.82	22.65	11
La Manche	29.21	22.46	26
St Omer	22.40	9.53	5

Total cases = 42
Missing cases = 0
Test of signficance, p=.2567, applying analysis of variance

The pattern of service delivery in La Manche is different from that in the other two areas. There are more separate home help services and

Table A.24. Means of hours per month of informal help with household tasks by area at time three

	Mean	Std dev	Cases
For all areas	29.69	15.47	29
Athis Mons	28.44	17.94	9
La Manche	29.19	14.92	16
St Omer	34.50	15.00	4

Total cases = 29
Missing cases = 0
Test of signficance, p=.8055, applying analysis of variance

Table A.25. Means of hours per month of informal help with nutrition by area at time two

	Mean	Std dev	Cases
For all areas	36.54	19.54	58
Athis Mons	44.91	28.14	11
La Manche	35.50	16.08	39
St Omer	30.13	20.27	8

Total cases = 58
Missing cases = 0
Test of signficance, p=.2270, applying analysis of variance

Table A.26. Means of hours per month of informal help with nutrition by area at time three

	Mean	Std dev	Cases
For all areas	42.58	21.32	36
Athis Mons	54.25	39.91	8
La Manche	38.21	11.49	24
St Omer	45.50	7.00	4

Total cases = 36
Missing cases = 0
Test of signficance, p=.1776, applying analysis of variance

Table A.27. Means of hours per month of informal help with shopping by area at time two

	Mean	*Std dev*	*Cases*
For all areas	17.14	12.36	74
Athis Mons	11.59	6.15	22
La Manche	20.79	13.38	43
St Omer	13.22	13.51	9

Total cases = 74
Missing cases = 0
Test of signficance, p=.0089, applying analysis of variance

Table A.28. Means of hours per month of informal help with shopping by area at time three

	Mean	*Std dev*	*Cases*
For all areas	18.87	15.37	50
Athis Mons	10.37	6.19	17
La Manche	21.84	16.64	29
St Omer	33.50	17.00	4

Total cases = 50
Missing cases = 0
Test of signficance, p=.0050, applying analysis of variance

infirmières libérales (self-employed nurses). In Athis Mons and St Omer, there are integrated models of service provision.

A.9. Synopsis

The main conclusions are summarised for (i) attrition and location; (ii) levels of input of help by informal caregivers; and (iii) levels of input from formal care agencies.

Table A.29. INSERM need category and presence of informal help with any task at time two: proportions of persons by area

		Yes	Total
Athis Mons			
Group 4	row %	60.0	100.0
	col %	12.0	
	no.	3	5
Group 3	row %	66.7	100.0
	col %	24.0	
	no.	6	9
Group 2	row %	88.9	100.0
	col %	64.0	
	no.	16	18
Total	row %	78.1	100.0
	col %	100.0	
	no.	25	32
La Manche			
Group 4	row %	66.7	100.0
	col %	6.9	
	no.	2	3
Group 3	row %	40.0	100.0
	col %	6.9	
	no.	2	5
Group 2	row %	52.6	100.0
	col %	69.0	
	no.	20	38
Group 1	row %	100.0	100.0
	col %	17.2	
	no.	5	5
Total	row %	56.9	100.0
	col %	100.0	
	no.	29	51
St Omer			
Group 4	row %	100.0	100.0
	col %	14.8	
	no.	4	4
Group 3	row %	100.0	100.0
	col %	33.3	
	no.	9	9
Group 2	row %	100.0	100.0
	col %	51.9	
	no.	14	14
Total	row %	100.0	100.0
	col %	100.0	
	no.	27	27

A.9.1. Attrition and user location (Tables A.1 to A.8)

The sample presented a high rate of attrition over the eighteen month period of the study, with about one-third remaining in the community at the end of the period. Tables A.7 and A.8 show how differently the two measures of dependency used predict outcomes. The Isaacs and Neville interval need scale had a higher level of correlation with entry into some form of shelter-with-care and morbidity.

A.9.2. Levels of help by informal caregivers (Tables A.9 to A.28)

There is variation across areas in the tasks undertaken by informal helpers, La Manche having consistently the highest proportion of informal care for all tasks. The pattern remains similar through time. This is true for both the proportions of cases receiving help and the pattern of mean hours of informal help. Nevertheless, its variation is better studied within the models embodied in Chapter 6.

A.9.3. Formal help (Tables A.29 to A.48)

There is a clear positive correlation between dependency levels and formal help, indicating good targeting of formal services. There is a quick response of formal services to needs, and by the time of second assessment the pattern of service delivery is well established. Across areas, and because of differences in the use of the ACTP, La Manche remains a lower user of formal services. This is particularly true for the tasks of housework and shopping (Tables A.33, A.34, A.37 and A.38).

For those cases who do receive formal services, the tables suggest a diversity of allocation policies. La Manche in particular consistently has higher mean hours. St Omer and Athis Mons operate unified home nursing and home care services, while in La Manche nursing services come from the *infirmières libérales*, independent of home care services. Although it is difficult to be certain, the unified approach to service delivery could well suggest a more efficient use of resources.

Table A.30. INSERM need category and presence of formal help with any task at time three: proportions of persons by area

		Yes	Total
Athis Mons			
Group 4	row %	60.0	100.0
	col %	15.0	
	no.	3	5
Group 3	row %	66.7	100.0
	col %	30.0	
	no.	6	9
Group 2	row %	100.0	100.0
	col %	55.0	
	no.	11	11
Total	row %	80.0	100.0
	col %	100.0	
	no.	20	25
La Manche			
Group 4	row %	50.0	100.0
	col %	9.5	
	no.	2	4
Group 2	row %	51.7	100.0
	col %	71.4	
	no.	15	29
Group 1	row %	100.0	100.0
	col %	19.0	
	no.	4	4
Total	row %	56.8	100.0
	col %	100.0	
	no.	21	37
St Omer			
Group 4	row %	100.0	100.0
	col %	29.4	
	no.	5	5
Group 3	row %	100.0	100.0
	col %	29.4	
	no.	5	5
Group 2	row %	100.0	100.0
	col %	29.4	
	no.	5	5
Group 1	row %	100.0	100.0
	col %	11.8	
	no.	2	2
Total	row %	100.0	100.0
	col %	100.0	
	no.	17	17

Table A.31. Presence of formal help with personal care at time two: proportions of persons by area

		Yes	Total
Athis Mons	row %	50.0	100.0
	no.	16	32
La Manche	row %	41.2	100.0
	no.	21	51
St Omer	row %	48.1	100.0
	no.	13	27
Total	%	45.5	100.0
	no.	50	110

Tests of significance:
Difference between all 3 areas: p=.697, applying a Chi-square test.
Difference between each area and other areas individually:
Between Athis Mons and La Manche: p=.873, applying a t-test.
Between Athis Mons and St Omer: p=.981, applying a t-test.
Between La Manche and St Omer: p=.860, applying a t-test.

Table A.32. Presence of formal help with personal care at time three: proportions of persons by area

		Yes	Total
Athis Mons	row %	42.0	100.0
	no.	11	25
La Manche	row %	43.2	100.0
	no.	16	37
St Omer	row %	35.3	100.0
	no.	33	17
Total	%	41.8	100.0
	no.	33	79

Tests of significance:
Difference between all 3 areas: p=.828, applying a Chi-square test.
Difference between each area and other areas individually:
Between Athis Mons and La Manche: p=.954, applying a t-test.
Between Athis Mons and St Omer: p=.582, applying a t-test.

Table A.33. Presence of formal help with household tasks at time two: proportions of persons by area

		Yes	Total
Athis Mons	row %	50.0	100.0
	no.	16	32
La Manche	row %	41.2	100.0
	no.	21	51
St Omer	row %	81.5	100.0
	no.	22	27
Total	%	53.6	100.0
	no.	59	110

Tests of significance:
Difference between all 3 areas: p=.003, applying a Chi-square test.
Difference between each area and other areas individually:
Between Athis Mons and La Manche: p=.440, applying a t-test.
Between Athis Mons and St Omer: p=.010, applying a t-test.
Between La Manche and St Omer: p=.000, applying a t-test.

Table A.34. Presence of formal help with household tasks at time three: proportions of persons by area

		Yes	Total
Athis Mons	row %	60.0	100.0
	no.	15	25
La Manche	row %	51.4	100.0
	no.	19	37
St Omer	row %	76.5	100.0
	no.	13	17
Total	%	59.5	100.0
	no.	47	79

Tests of significance:
Difference between all 3 areas: p=.217, applying a Chi-square test.
Difference between each area and other areas individually:
Between Athis Mons and La Manche: p=.509, applying a t-test.
Between Athis Mons and St Omer: p=.266, applying a t-test.
Between La Manche and St Omer: p=.071, applying a t-test.

Table A.35. Presence of formal help with nutrition at time two: proportions of persons by area

		Yes	*Total*
Athis Mons	row %	25.0	100.0
	no.	8	32
La Manche	row %	15.7	100.0
	no.	8	51
St Omer	row %	25.9	100.0
	no.	7	27
Total	%	20.9	100.0
	no.	23	110

Tests of significance:
Difference between all 3 areas: p=.455, applying a Chi-square test.
Difference between each area and other areas individually:
Between Athis Mons and La Manche: p=.322, applying a t-test.
Between Athis Mons and St Omer: p=.937, applying a t-test.
Between La Manche and St Omer: p=.312, applying a t-test.

Table A.36. Presence of formal help with nutrition at time three: proportions of persons by area

		Yes	*Total*
Athis Mons	row %	24.0	100.0
	no.	6	25
La Manche	row %	29.7	100.0
	no.	11	37
St Omer	row %	0.0	100.0
	no.	0	17
Total	%	21.5	100.0
	no.	17	79

Tests of significance:
Difference between all 3 areas: p=.044, applying a Chi-square test.
Difference between each area and other areas individually:
Between Athis Mons and La Manche: p=.623, applying a t-test.
Between Athis Mons and St Omer: p=.011, applying a t-test.
Between La Manche and St Omer: p=.000, applying a t-test.

Table A.37. Presence of formal help with shopping at time two: proportions of persons by area

		Yes	Total
Athis Mons	row %	21.9	100.0
	no.	7	32
La Manche	row %	13.7	100.0
	no.	7	51
St Omer	row %	48.1	100.0
	no.	13	27
Total	%	24.5	100.0
	no.	27	110

Tests of significance:
Difference between all 3 areas: p=.003, applying a Chi-square test.
Difference between each area and other areas individually:
Between Athis Mons and La Manche: p=.363, applying a t-test.
Between Athis Mons and St Omer: p=.037, applying a t-test.
Between La Manche and St Omer: p=.003, applying a t-test.

Table A.38. Presence of formal help with shopping at time three: proportions of persons by area

		Yes	Total
Athis Mons	row %	28.0	100.0
	no.	7	25
La Manche	row %	18.9	100.0
	no.	7	37
St Omer	row %	41.2	100.0
	no.	7	17
Total	%	26.6	100.0
	no.	21	79

Tests of significance:
Difference between all 3 areas: p=.224, applying a Chi-square test.
Difference between each area and other areas individually:
Between Athis Mons and La Manche: p=.424, applying a t-test.
Between Athis Mons and St Omer: p=.397, applying a t-test.
Between La Manche and St Omer: p=.122, applying a t-test.

Table A.39. Means of hours per month of formal help with any task by area at time two

	Mean	Std dev	Cases
For all areas	53.60	67.15	81
Athis Mons	54.59	66.18	25
La Manche	69.47	84.75	29
St Omer	35.63	38.53	27

Total cases = 81
Missing cases = 0
Test of signficance, p=.1695, applying analysis of variance

Table A.40. Means of hours per month of formal help with any task by area at time three

	Mean	Std dev	Cases
For all areas	66.39	102.63	58
Athis Mons	53.08	59.79	20
La Manche	110.76	151.14	21
St Omer	27.24	17.06	17

Total cases = 58
Missing cases = 0
Test of signficance, p=.0315, applying analysis of variance

Table A.41. Means of hours per month of formal help with personal care by area at time two

	Mean	Std dev	Cases
For all areas	25.45	24.54	50
Athis Mons	22.92	15.21	16
La Manche	32.92	31.19	21
St Omer	16.49	18.87	13

Total cases = 50
Missing cases = 0
Test of signficance, p=.1462, applying analysis of variance

Table A.42. Means of hours per month of formal help with personal care by area at time three

	Mean	*Std dev*	*Cases*
For all areas	27.59	19.69	33
Athis Mons	19.88	8.55	11
La Manche	36.35	23.74	16
St Omer	18.33	12.85	6

Total cases = 33
Missing cases = 0
Test of signficance, p=.0399, applying analysis of variance

Table A.43. Means of hours per month of formal help with household tasks by area at time two

	Mean	*Std dev*	*Cases*
For all areas	21.09	14.23	59
Athis Mons	16.94	9.56	16
La Manche	22.92	13.58	21
St Omer	22.36	17.33	22

Total cases = 59
Missing cases = 0
Test of signficance, p=.3961, applying analysis of variance

Table A.44. Means of hours per month of formal help with household tasks by area at time three

	Mean	*Std dev*	*Cases*
For all areas	20.43	10.63	47
Athis Mons	19.59	11.21	15
La Manche	24.00	11.72	19
St Omer	16.18	6.34	13

Total cases = 47
Missing cases = 0
Test of signficance, p=.1149, applying analysis of variance

Table A.45. Means of hours per month of formal help with nutrition by area at time two

	Mean	*Std dev*	*Cases*
For all areas	28.99	38.56	23
Athis Mons	45.00	61.65	8
La Manche	25.63	15.40	8
St Omer	14.52	11.85	7

Total cases = 23
Missing cases = 0
Test of signficance, p=.3110, applying analysis of variance

Table A.46. Means of hours per month of formal help with nutrition by area at time three

	Mean	*Std dev*	*Cases*
For all areas	35.41	19.67	17
Athis Mons	36.33	26.49	6
La Manche	34.91	16.36	11
St Omer			0

Total cases = 17
Missing cases = 0
Test of signficance, p=.8919, applying analysis of variance

Table A.47. Means of hours per month of formal help with shopping by area at time two

	Mean	*Std dev*	*Cases*
For all areas	9.07	7.71	27
Athis Mons	5.00	2.34	7
La Manche	9.71	9.48	7
St Omer	10.92	8.23	13

Total cases = 27
Missing cases = 0
Test of signficance, p=.2615, applying analysis of variance

Table A.48. Means of hours per month of formal help with shopping by area at time three

	Mean	*Std dev*	*Cases*
For all areas	8.09	9.01	21
Athis Mons	5.54	1.82	7
La Manche	14.14	14.15	7
St Omer	4.57	1.51	7

Total cases = 21
Missing cases = 0
Test of signficance, p=.0852, applying analysis of variance

Glossary

G.1. An explanation of terms used in the text

G.1.1. France

Aide sociale. Income support for those who lack the means to access health or welfare benefits covered by the *régime générale*. Thus, in the context of this report, it pays for home help inputs where this is not available through other entitlement.

Allocation compensatrice pour tierce personne (ACTP). A cash allowance paid after assessment of dependency and financial means test, by the *départements*. The upper level is paid according to a nationally determined level, but the allowance, which was intended for physically handicappped adults, is applied according to local policy criteria established by each *département's conseil général*. This is to be gradually replaced by an allowance specifically for older people, the *prestation spécifique dépendance (PSD)*, from 1 January 1997 (see Box 2 in Chapter 3).

Association: A not-for profit organisation covered by the terms of the Law of 1901. Most forms of home care service are of this type, including *association mandataire*, which acts as an agent for the elderly person to enable them to employ trained home care staff while retaining the entitlement to fiscal benefits intended for those directly employing private help.

Caisses. A general term covering many types of financial institutions. Normally means the state social security funds such as: *Caisse nationale d'assurance maladie* (CNAM), the health insurance fund, organised via regional centres (*Caisses régionales d'assurance maladie*, CRAM) and local offices (*Caisses primaires d'assurance maladie*, CPAM). The CRAM is the level which determines local application of national policy, for example determining the level of per capita funding for home nursing services (*services de soins*).

Caisse nationale d'assurance vieillesse des travailleurs salariés (CNAVTS or, often, CNAV). the main pension fund, covering all those in employment, other than those such as government staff, railways employees, etc., whose fund offers equal or better coverage to what is known as the *régime générale*. Through CNAV's *action sociale* branch, it pays for home care of a social support nature. At regional level and below, it functions via the offices of *assurance maladie* and so at those levels it is often known undifferentiatedly as CRAM or CPAM, although in fact it is a separate entity.

Chèque service/chèque autonomie. (Also known as the *chèque emploi-service*). A system designed to facilitate direct payment of wages to a domestic employee, whereby the employer can buy through the post office or bank cheques which include the appropriate social security contributions, the employee receiving repayment of their full hourly rate as shown on the cheque, the employer paying the hourly rate plus the social contributions. They can currently be used for a maximum of eight hours worked per week, or one full month's work per annum, although these limits are to be increased.

Commune. Lowest administrative level of French government, headed by a *maire*, who combines the role of elected representative and local agent of the state with emergency powers which can be delegated by the *préfét*. Has considerably more autonomy than the English equivalent, the parish council.

Conseil général. Elected council for the *département*.

Département. A tier of local governement which in size approximates to the new English unitary authorities. Responsible for planning and supervision of social services.

Mutualités. Private mutual funds which top up the basic cover offered through the *régime général*. Thus, the state insurance, CRAM, will refund up to 75 per cent of the cost of prescribed medicines, and a *mutualité* would cover the cost of the balance. A further example of a *mutualité* is the *mutualité sociale agricole* (MSA), which in fact forms part of the basic insurance structure, like the *caisses nationales*, but only for farmers and related employment groups.

Obligation alimentaire. A requirement under article 213 and 215 et seq of the Civil Code for members of a family to provide help to each other. In terms of care of the elderly, it places an obligation on spouse, ascendents and descendents, such as grandchildren, or son- or daugther-in-law, to pay for the elderly relative if they enter institutional care and would be at the financial level of *aide sociale.* However, it does not apply to the cost of home help where paid for by aide sociale or ACTP, or to the daily charge for 'hotel' costs for hospital inpatient stays. There is no researched evidence as to its effects.

Préfet. The representation of the state administration at the level of the *région* or *département.*

Régime générale. Main state insurance scheme covering health and pensions (*Caisse nationale d'assurance maladie* or *Caisse nationale d'assurance vieillesse*).

Régimes complémentaire. Not-for-profit insurance schemes that supplement the *régime générale.* There are several independent *caisses,* usually described by their collective association: *Association des régimes de retraite complémentaire* (ARRCO).

Régimes spéciaux. For those in state employment, an insurance scheme which provides the equal or better of the state *régime générale.*

Région. Tier of local governement above the *département,* normally covering two to four such *départements.* Their role in social services is mainly one of coordination, particularly in matters of standard-setting.

G.1.2. England

Attendance allowance. A cash allowance paid by the Department of Social Security intended to cover some of the costs associated with disability. It is paid at two levels for the elderly, the lower being for those needing help during the day, the higher for those needing help

Box G.1. *Concentration of responsibility, authority and financing: services and their financing agencies for social and nursing care in England and France*

Category	*England & Wales*	*Service*	*France*
	Financing agency		*Financing agency*
Cash benefits	Central government	Attendance allowance, invalid care allowance – allocation compensatrice (ACTP) Prestation spécifique dépendance (PSD)	Conseils généraux
Benefits in kind *Persons living in private households* Social care	SSD User	Home help – aide ménagère	Régime général ARRCO Aide sociale User
		Care worker – garde à domicile, soins à domicile	CNAVTS CNAM Aide sociale
		Meals-on-wheels – repas à domicile	Commune User
		Day centre – centre de jour	Régime général ARRCO Conseil général Commune User

Box G.1. Continued

<table>
<tr><td rowspan="2">Health care</td><td rowspan="2">Health</td><td>Nursing auxiliary</td><td>CNAM
Aide sociale</td></tr>
<tr><td>District nurse – infirmière libérale, soins à domicile</td><td>CNAM
User</td></tr>
<tr><td rowspan="2">Persons living in shelter with care
Social care</td><td rowspan="2">SSD
User</td><td>Short-term care – court séjour, soins répit</td><td rowspan="2">User
Family
Aide sociale</td></tr>
<tr><td>Long-term residential home – maison de retraite</td></tr>
<tr><td rowspan="2">Social with nursing care</td><td>SSD
Health
User</td><td>Nursing home – maison de retraite avec section cure médicale</td><td rowspan="2">User
Family under obligation alimentaire
Aide sociale
CNAM</td></tr>
<tr><td>Health</td><td>Long-stay hospital – hôpital long séjour</td></tr>
</table>

both night and day. It is set at a level which corresponds to about half that of its nearest French equivalent, ACTP, but it is not means-tested.

County council. Level of local authority responsible for social services, except in urban areas, where this role is taken by borough councils. Is equal in size to two to three French *départements*. Areas of action include planning, coordination, assessment and, although decreasingly, service provision.

Department of Health. Ministry of central government responsible for running the National Health Service and also determining policy for social services departments of local government authorities. It further influences local social services through its monitoring role, carried out by its Social Services Inspectorate (SSI), and through research which it funds.

Department of Social Security. Central government ministry responsible for paying state benefits and allowances.

District council. Lowest tier of local goverment that has significant executive functions, mainly to do with housing and planning. Some six or more district councils would constitute a county council area.

Unitary authority. Currently being set up as a result of the 1994/5 local government review, some areas are seeing their county and district councils being abolished, to be replaced by unitary authorities which group together two or three district councils and take over responsibility for the full range of local authority tasks, including housing and social services.

G.2. List of variables used in modelling

G.2.1. The French data

ACTP	Level of ACTP received
AFOR	Formal help for companionship
ALZ	Alzheimer's disease
AREA1	Area 1: La Manche
BBOUND	Bedbound
BEHAV	Disturbed behaviour
CANC	Cancer
CIRC	Circulatory problems
CLOFEM	Helper is close female relative
DISAB	Quasi-input weighted index of disability
DISHOUS	Disability (DISAB) x help for housework
ENTRY	Entry into institutional care
FORPCT	Formal help for personal care
HBOUND	Housebound
HIGHPCEXP	Cost of inputs for personal care tasks greater than half the cost of residential care
HINF	Informal help for housework
HNO	Number in household
HOME	User lives in own home
INCONT	Faecal and/or urinary incontinence
INFHOA	Informal helper comes within scope of the *obligation alimentaire*
INFMEAL	Informal help with meals
INFPCT	Informal help with personal care
INSERM	INSERM disability level
ISAAC	Isaacs & Neville disability level
LIVCH	User lives near their children
MALE	User is male
MARRID	User is married
MFOR	Formal help with meals
RESP	Respiratory problems
SFOR	Formal help for shopping
SINF	Informal help for shopping
SKEL	Musculo-skeletal problems

SUITA	Suitability of accommodation
VIS	Visual impairment
WANDER	User has tendency to wander

G.2.2. The English data

ACOST2	Average cost of social services input to household
ACOST3	Total average cost of all inputs to household
ALL&ANG	User receives attendance allowance and carer expresses feeling of anger towards user
ALLHTIME	Minutes spent on housework by all carers
ALLSTIME	Minutes spent on social work by all carers
BBOUND	User is bedbound
CARAIDF	Carer helps user financially
CAREANG	Carer expresses feelings of anger towards user
CARHOSP	Carer has recently been in hospital
CARMALE	Carer is male
CONFUSED	User suffers from confusion
COST	Average cost of formal services to user
COTHPER	Person close to carer died recently
DEATHSP	Spouse of user died recently
DISAB	Quasi-input weighted index of disability
ENTRY	Entry into institutional care
EPAIDF	User helps carer financially
EPWANDER	User has tendency to wander
FAECAL	Faecal incontinence
FREQVSTS	Frequency of carer's visits to user
HBENEFIT	Household receives housing benefit
HEATING	Presence of central heating
HHATTENT	Household receives attendence allowance
HHRPENSN	Household receives retirement pension
INCOME	Household income index
INCOME2	INCOME squared
INFHELP	Presence of informal help
LONGVST	Length of carer's visit
LOVEAFF	Carer's reason for caring is through love and affection

MAL&ALO	User is male and lives alone
MALE	User is male
PET	User has a pet
RWDCARE	Carer finds caring for user rewarding
SINGLE	User is single
SSDCMPNY	Social services provide help with company
SSDHWORK	Social services provide help with housework
SSDMEALS	Social services provide help with meals
SSDPCARE	Social services provide help with personal care
SSDSHOPS	Social services provide help with shopping
TASKTIME	Time spent on all tasks by different carers
TIME2	Second data collection round
URIN	Urinary incontinence
WALKAID	User needs walking aid

References

Abrams, P. (1977) Community care: some research problems and priorities, *Policy and Politics*, 6, 125-52.

Arfeux-Vaucher, G. (1986) *Les beneficiaries âgées de l'allocation compensatrice*, Fondation nationale de gérontologie, Paris.

Arrow, K.J. (1972) Gifts and exchanges, *Philosophy and Public Affairs*, 1, 343-62.

Assemblé nationale (1991) *Rapport d'information déposé en application de l'article 145 du réglement par la commission des affaires culturelles famiales et sociales sur les personnes âgées dépendantes: Vivre Ensemble: le Rapport Boulard*, Automédon, Paris.

Association of Directors of Social Services (ADSS) (1982) *Report of the Second Survey of the Extent and Effects of Cuts/Savings in Expenditure on the Personal Social Services*, ADSS, Newcastle upon Tyne.

Attias-Donfut, C. and Rozenkier, A. (1981) *Etudes et recherche: Vieillir chez soi: I. Les bénéficiaires*, Caisse nationale de l'assurance vieillesse, Paris.

Attias-Donfut, C., Renaut, S. and Rozenkier, A. (1994) Vie à domicile et aide bénévole, *Gerontologie et sociéte*, 71, 150-60.

Audit Commission (1985) *Managing Social Services for the Elderly More Effectively*, HMSO, London.

Audit Commission (1986) *Making a Reality of Community Care*, HMSO, London.

Audit Commission (1987) Balancing the care equation: progress with community care, *Community Care Bulletin Number 3*, March 1996.

Baldock, J. and Evers, A. (1992) Innovations and care of the elderly: the cutting edge of change for social welfare systems. Examples from Sweden, the Netherlands and the United Kingdom, *Ageing and Society*, 12, 3, 289-312.

Balladur, E. (1995) *La Lettre Eurosenior*, 8, May, tertio en partenariat avec CERIS, Paris.

Banerjee, S., Shamash, K., Macdonald, A.J.D. and Mann, A.H. (1996) Randomised controlled trial of effect of intervention by psychogeriatric team on depression in frail elderly people at home, *British Medical Journal*, 313, 7064, 1058-61.

Bebbington, A.C. and Davies, B.P. (1983) Equity and efficiency in the allocation of the personal social services, *Journal of Social Policy*, 12, 3, 309-30.

Bezat, J.-M. (1995) La 'prestation autonomie' pour les personnes âgées vivant à domicile entrera en vigueur début 1996, *Le Monde*, 6 July.

Bouget, D., Tartarin, R., Frossard, M. and Tripier, P. (eds) (1990) *Le Prix de la Dépendance: comparison des dépenses des personnes âgées selon leur mode d'hébergement*, La Documentation Française, Paris.

Bradshaw, J. (1988) Welfare benefits, in R. Walker and G. Parker (eds) *Money Matters: Income, Wealth and Financial Welfare*, Sage, London.

Braun, T. and Stourm, M. (1988) *Les Personnes Âgées Dépendantes: Rapport au Secrétaire d'Etat chargé de la sécurité sociale*, La Documentation Française, Paris.

Brody, E. and Brody, S. (1985) The informal system of health care, in C. Eisdorfer (ed.) *Reshaping Health Care for the Elderly: Recommendations for National Policy*, Johns Hopkins University Press, Baltimore, Maryland.

Cantor, M.H. (1980) The informal support system: its relevance in the lives of the elderly, in E. Borgotta and N. McClusky (eds) Aging and Society. Sage, Beverley Hills, California.

Capitman, J. (1994) Targeting community care, *The Gerontologist*, 34, 580-81.

Challis, D. and Davies, B.P. (1981) Community care projects: costs and effectiveness, in J.C. Henrard (ed.) *Les Colloques d'INSERM, vol. 10*, INSERM, Paris.

Challis, D., Darton, R., Johnson, L., Stone, M. and Traske, K. (1991) An evaluation of an alternative to hospital care for frail elderly patients: I. The model of care, *Age and Ageing*, 20, 236-44.

Challis, D., Darton, R., Johnson, L., Stone, M. and Traske, K. (1994) *Case Management in a Geriatric Setting: The Darlington Community Care Project*, Ashgate, Aldershot.

Chirac, J. (1995) *La Lettre Eurosenior*, 8, May, tertio en partenariat avec CERIS, Paris.

Chombeau, C. (1992) Le projet du gouvernement sur les personnes âgées dépendantes, *Le Monde*, 22 December, 10.

Colvez, A. (1997) Le programme d'action et d'évaluation gérontologique de Lunel: quels enseignements pour une coordination efficace des prestations aux personnes âgées dépendantes? *Revue Française des Affaires Sociales: Numéro Hors-Série: Le vieillissement comme une processus*, Federation CRI, ORS, INSERM and VISA, Paris.

Colvez, A., Varnoux, N. and Bouquet, G. (1985) *Differences régionales de l'état de santé des personnes agées vivant à domicile*, INSERM Unité 164, Paris.

Colvez, A., Dhivert, J.-C., Puech, O. and Ribera, J. (1995) *Prevention de la dépendance: programme d'action et d'évaluation gérontologiques dans le bassin de vie de Lunel*, Féderation CRI ORS INSERM et VISA, Montpelier, France.

Commissariat général du plan (1981) *Vieillir demain*, The Lion Report, La Documentation Française, Paris.

Commissariat général du plan (1991) *Dépendance et Solidarités Mieux Aider les Personnes Agées: Rapport de la Commission presidée par Pierre Schopflin*, La Documentation Française, Paris.

Coopers and Lybrand Consulting Group (1994) *Home Care Client Classification (HCC) System, Final Report*, Alberta Health, Alberta.

Curtis, S. (1986) *Home Help Provision to the Elderly in France and England: A National and Metropolitan Comparison*, Department of Geography and Earth Science, Queen Mary College, London.

Curtis, S., Bucquet, D. and Colvez, A. (1992) Sources of instrumental support for dependent elderly people in three parts of France, *Ageing and Society*, 12, 329-54.

Davies, B.P. (1968) *Social Needs and Resources in Local Services*, Michael Joseph, London.

Davies, B.P. (1974) Proposal for a Kent Community Care Project, Kent Community Care Project Paper 1, Personal Social Service Research Unit, University of Kent, Canterbury.

Davies, B.P. (1978) *Universality, Selectivity and Effectiveness in Social Policy*, Heinemann, London.

Davies, B.P. (1981) Strategic goals and piecemeal innovations: adjusting to the new balance of needs and resources, in E. Goldberg and S. Hatch (eds) *A New Look at the Personal Social Services*, Policy Studies Institute, London.

Davies, B.P. (1986) American lessons for British policy and research on long-term care of the elderly, *Quarterly Journal of Social Affairs*, 2, 3, 321-55.

Davies, B.P. (1988) Making a reality of community care: a critique of the Audit Commission's Report, *British Journal of Social Work*, 18, supplement, 1-11.

Davies, B.P. (1989) Case management in the UK: current debate and future prospects, Discussion Paper 672, Personal Social Services Research Unit, University of Kent, Canterbury.

Davies, B.P. (1990) Why we must fight the eighth deadly sin: parochialism, *Journal of Aging and Social Policy*, 1, 217-36.

Davies, B.P. (1992) *Case Management, Equity and Efficiency: The International Experience*, Personal Social Services Research Unit, University of Kent, Canterbury.

Davies, B.P. (1993) Caring for the frail elderly: an international perspective, *Generations*, 17, 4, 51-55.

Davies, B.P. (1994) Improving the case management process, in OECD, *Caring for the Frail Elderly: New Directions for Change*, OECD, Paris.

Davies, B.P. (1998) Shelter with care and the community care reforms, in R. Jack (ed.) *Institutions in Community Care*, Macmillan, London.

Davies, B.P. and Baines, B. (1994) Attitudes to residential care and the subsequent probability of admission: analysis of a new cohort of recipients of community-based services, in D.J. Challis, B.P. Davies and K. Traske (eds) *Community Care: New Agenda and the Challenges for the UK and Overseas*, Avebury, Aldershot.

Davies, B.P. and Challis, D.J. (1981) A production relations evaluation of the meeting of needs in the Community Care Projects, in E.M. Goldberg and N. Connelly (eds) *Evaluative Research in Social Care*, Heinemann, London.

Davies, B.P. and Challis, D.J. (1986) *Matching Resources to Needs in Community Care*, Gower, Aldershot.

Davies, B.P. and Chesterman, J. (1998) *Budget-holding Case Management in Two Routine Programmes*, Ashgate, Aldershot, forthcoming.

Davies, B.P. and Fernández, J.L. (1997) On the sensitivity of proportions of SSD recipients of community social services excluded and costs to variations in qualifying levels of eligibility, Discussion Paper 1341, Personal Social Services Research Unit, University of Kent, Canterbury.

Davies, B.P. and Knapp, M.R. (1981) *Old People's Homes and the Production of Welfare*. Routledge and Kegan Paul, London.

Davies, B.P., Bebbington, A.C., Charnley, H. in collaboration with Baines, B., Ferlie, E., Hughes, M. and Twigg, J. (1990) *Resources, Needs and Outcomes in Community-Based Care: A comparative study of the production of welfare for elderly persons in ten local authorities in England and Wales*, PSSRU studies, Avebury/Gower, Aldershot.

Davies, B.P., Fernández, J.L. and Saunders, R. (1995a) Substitution between informal and formal care inputs and the probability of entry to institutions for long-term care among elderly people receiving home care service in England and France, Discussion Paper 1155, Personal Social Services Research Unit, University of Kent, Canterbury.

Davies, B.P., Warburton, R.W. and Fernández, J. (1995b) Do different case management approaches affect who gets what? Preliminary results from a comparative British study, *Care Plan*, December, 26-7.

Davies, B.P., Fernández, J.L. and Warburton, R.W. (1996a) Post-reform community care for elderly people: who gets how much of what service?, *Care Plan*, 3, 2, December, 25-30.

Davies, B.P., Fernández, J.L. and Warburton, R.W. (1996b) Evaluating community care, Discussion Paper 1226, Personal Social Services Research Unit, University of Kent, Canterbury.

Davies, B.P., Warburton, R.W. and Fernández, J.L. (1996c) Care management, other community care costs, needs and outcomes, *Hong Kong Journal of Gerontology*, 10, supplement, 255-259.

Davies, B.P., Fernández, J.L. and Saunders, R. (1997) *Needs, Processes and Service Packages: Post-Reform Community Care at the Case Level*, Personal Social Services Research Unit, University of Kent, Canterbury.

De Lew, N., Greenberg, G. and Kinchen, K. (1992) A layman's guide to the US health care system, *Health Care Financing Review*, Fall, 14, 1, 151-170.

Department of Health (1990) *Community Care in the Next Decade and Beyond, Policy Guidance*, HMSO, London.

Department of Health (1997a) *Community Care Statistics 1996 — Statistics Bulletin 1*, Department of Health, London.

Department of Health (1997b) *Statistical Bulletin: Residential Accommodation*, Department of Health, London.

Department of Health and Social Security (1974) *Social Security Provision for Chronically Sick and Disabled Persons*, HC 276, DHSS, London.
Department of Health and Social Security, SSI (1987) From Home Help to Home Care: An Analysis of Policy, Resourcing and Service Management, HMSO, London.
Department of Social Security (1993) *Statistics*, HMSO, London.
Esping-Andersen, G. (1990) *The Three Worlds of Welfare Capitalism*, Princeton University Press, Princeton.
Evandrou, M. and Winter, D. (1988) *The Distribution of Domiciliary and Primary Health Care in Britain*, STICERD, London School of Economics, London.
Evans, M., Paugram, S. and Prélis, J. (1995) *Chunnel Vision: Poverty, Social Exclusion and the Debate on Social Welfare in France and Britain*, STICERD, London School of Economics, London.
Evers, A. (1994) Shared challenges, different responses: the future of services for elderly people in increasingly mixed and pluralistic welfare systems, in D.J. Challis, B.P. Davies and K. Traske (eds) *Community Care: New Agendas and Challenges from the UK and Overseas*, Arena, Aldershot.
Evers, A. and Svetlik, I. (1993) *New Welfare Mixes in Care for the Elderly, Vol. 3, Canada, France, Germany, Italy, UK*, European Centre Social Welfare Policy and Research, Vienna.
Evers, A. and van der Zanden, G. (1993) *Better Care for Dependent People Living at Home*, Netherlands Institute of Gerontology, Bunnik.
Fondation de France (1992) *Une vieille idée pleine d'avenir*, Study day on *La coordination gérontologique*, March, Fondation de France, Paris.
Forder, J., Knapp, M.R. and Wistow, G (1996) Competition in the mixed economy of care, *Journal of Social Policy*, 25, 2, 201-21.
Fowler, N. (1984) Buxton speech to Joint Council of Social Services.
Friend, J.K. and Jessup, L.G. (1969) *Local Government and Strategic Choice*, Tavistock, London.
Goldberg, E.M. and Connelly, N. (1982) *The Effectiveness of Social Care for the Elderly*, Heineman, London.
Goldberg, E.M. and Warburton, R.W. (1979) *Ends and Means in Social Work*, Allen and Unwin, London.
Gouriou, J. (1993) La prestation de garde à domicile créé par la caisse nationale d'assurance vieillesse en 1992, *Retraite et Sociéte*, 3.

Greene, V., Lovely, M.E. and Ondrich, J.I. (1993) The cost-effectiveness of community services in a frail elderly population, *The Gerontologist*, 33, 177-90.

Griffiths, R. (1988) *Community Care: Agenda for Action*, HMSO, London.

Guillemard, A.-M. (1986) *Le declin du social: formation et crise des politiques de la vieillesse*, Presses Universitaire de France, Paris.

Guillemard, A.-M. and Frossard, M. (1993) Risks and achievements in strengthening home care: France, in A. Evers and G.H. van der Zanden (eds) *Better Care for Dependent People Living at Home: Meeting the Agenda in Services for the Elderly*, NIG, Bunnik, The Netherlands.

Gwynne, W.D. and Fean, L. (1978) *Home Help Services in Cumbria*, Cumbria Social Services Department.

Habib, K. and Windmiller, K. (1992) Family support to elderly persons in Israel, in H.L. Kendig (ed.) *Family Support for the Elderly: The International Experience*, Oxford University Press, Oxford.

Henrard, J.C. (1992) *Les systèmes d'aides aux personnes âgées*, La Documentation Française, Paris.

Henrard, J.C. (1994) Financing care for elderly people in the European Community, in D.J. Challis, B.P. Davies and K. Traske (eds) *Community Care: New Agendas and Challenges from the UK and Overseas*, Arena, Aldershot.

Henrard, J.C. and Ankri, J. (1994) Les prestations du secteur médico-social, *Gerontologie et Societe*, 71, 110-22.

Henrard, J.C., Cassou, B. and Le Disert, D. (1990) The effects of system characteristics on policy implementation and functioning of care for the elderly in France, *International Journal of Health Services*, 20, 125-39.

Henrard, J.C., Ankri, J. and Isnard, M.-C. (1991) Home care services in France, in A. Jamieson (ed.) *Home Care for Older People in Europe: A Comparison of Policies and Practices*, Oxford University Press, Oxford.

Hirsch, F. (1977) *Social Limits to Growth*, Routledge and Kegan Paul, Henley-on-Thames.

Hosmer, D.W. and Lemeshow, S. (1989) *Applied Logistic Regression*, John Wiley, New York.

Hunt, A. (1973) *The Home Help Service in England and Wales*, HMSO, London.

Isaacs, B. and Neville, Y. (1975) *The Measurement of Need in Old People*, Scottish Home and Health Department, HMSO, London.

Jette, A.M., Tennstedt, S. and Crawford, S. (1995) How does formal and informal community care affect nursing home use, *Journal of Gerontology*, 54, 508-12.

Joel, M. and Martin, C. (1994) Payment for care: the case of France, in A. Evers, M. Pijl and C. Ungerson (eds) *Payments for Care: A Comparative Overview*, Avebury, Aldershot.

Johnston, J. (1963) *Econometric Methods*, McGraw Hill, New York.

Joseph Rowntree Foundation Inquiry (1996) *Meeting the Costs of Continuing Care*, Joseph Rowntree Foundation, York.

Jourdain, A. (1996) *La prestation expérimentale dépendance en Ille et Vilaine*, Ecole Nationale de la Santé Publique, Rennes.

Judge, K. and Matthews, J. (1980) *Charging for Social Care: A Study of Consumer Charges and the Personal Social Services*, Allen & Unwin, London.

Kane, R.A. (1988) The noblest experiment of them all: learning from the national chanelling evaluation, *Health Services Research*, 23, 189-98.

Kane, R.L., Kane, R.A., Finch, M., Harrington, C., Newcomer, R., Miller, N. and Hulbert, M. (1987) S/HMOs, the second generation: building on the experience of the first social health maintenance organization demonstrations, *Journal of the American Geriatrics Society*, 45, 101-107.

Kassner, E. and Williams, L. (1997) *Taking Care of their Own: State-Funded Home and Community-Based Care Programs for Older Persons*, Public Policy Institute, American Association of Retired People, Washington, DC.

Kemper, P., Murtaugh, C. and Spillman, B.C. (1991) A lifetime perspective on proposals for financing nursing home care, *Inquiry*, 28, 333-444.

Kendall, J. and Knapp, M.R. (1995) *The Voluntary Sector in the UK*, Manchester University Press, Manchester.

Klein, R. and O'Higgins, M. (1985) Social policy after incrementalism, in R. Klein and M. O'Higgins (eds) *The Future of Welfare*, Basil Blackwell, Oxford.

Knapp, M.R. (1984) *The Economics of Social Care*, Macmillan, London.

Kraan, R.J., Baldock, J., Davies, B.P., Evers, A., Johansson, L., Knapen, M., Thorslund, M. and Tunissen, C. (1991) *Care for the Elderly: Significant Innovations in Three European Countries*, Campus Westview, Frankfurt and New York.

Inspection Générale des Affaires Sociales (1962) *Rapport sur la dependance des personnes agées* (The Laroque report), La Documentation Française, Paris.

Laing & Buisson (1994) *Community Care Market News*, 1, 8.

Le Disert, D., di Palma, M., Leonard, M.-C., Henrard, J.C., Cassou, B. and Ankri, J. (1989) Caracteristiques du reseau social et du support occasionnel des personnes âgées de 75 et plus, *Gérontologie et société*, 48, 58-67.

Leach, E. (1971) The heart of the matter: a review of *The Gift Relationship*, *New Society*, 21 January.

Leat, D. (1988) *The Role of Social Security Payments in Encouraging Non-Kin to Take Caring Responsibilities*, Department of Sociology, University of Warwick, Coventry.

Les Dossiers de l'ADEPHA (1997) Association des Directeurs d'Etablissements d'Hébergement pour Personnes Agées (ADEPHA), January, Paris.

Linsk, N.L., Keigher, S.M., Simon-Rusinowitz, L. and England, S.E. (1992) *Wages for Caring and Compensating Family Care of the Elderly*, Praeger, Westport, Connecticut.

Manton, K.G. and Stallard, E. (1992) Analysis of underwriting factors for AAPCC, *Health Care Financing Review*, Fall, 14, 1, 117-132.

Ministry of Social Affairs and National Solidarity (1986) Circulaire No. 86-14, 7 March, Paris.

Moreland Commission (1975) *Federal Policy and the Growth of the Industry to 1975: The Creation and Growth of a Frankenstein*, New York State Moreland Act Commission on Nursing Homes and Residential Facilities, Albany, New York.

O'Keefe, J. (1996) *Determining the Need for Long-Term Care Services: An Analysis of Health and Functional Eligibility Criteria in Medicaid Home and Community-Based Waiver Programs*, Public Policy Institute, AARP, Washington, DC.

Olson, P. (1993) Caregiving and long-term health care in the People's Republic of China, *Journal of Aging and Social Policy*, 5, 91-110.

Organisation for Economic Cooperation and Development (OECD) (1994) *Caring for Frail Elderly People: New Directions in Care*, OECD, Paris, France.

Organisation for Economic Cooperation and Development (OECD) (1996) *Caring for Frail Elderly People: Policies in Evolution*, Social Policy Studies 19, OECD, Paris.

ORSMIP (1993) *Le Bulletin, Numéro Spécial Personnes Agées*, 31, September.

Piktialis, D.S. (1981) *Case Management and Policy Development in Massachusetts*, Department of Elder Affairs, State of Massachusetts, Boston, Massachusetts.

Pollitt, C. (1990) *Managerialism and the Public Services: The Anglo-American Experience*, Blackwell, Oxford.

Puech, O. and Colvez, A. (1995) *Targeting Services to Disabled Elderly*, INSERM, Montpelier.

Qureshi, H. (1990) The hierarchy of obligations among informal carers, *Ageing and Society*, 10, 455-58.

Qureshi, H. and Walker, A. (1989) *The Caring Relationship*, Macmillan, Basingstoke.

Qureshi, H., Challis, D.J. and Davies, B.P. (1989) *Helpers in Case-Managed Community Care*, Gower, Aldershot.

Revue Française des Affaires Sociales (1997) *Numéro Hors-Série: Le vieillissement comune processus*, Federation CRI, ORS, INSERM and VISA, Paris.

Richards, E. (1996) *Paying for Long-Term Care*, Institute for Public Policy Research and London Economics, London.

Ridley, N. (1988) *The Local Right: Enabling not Providing*, Policy Study No. 92, Centre for Policy Studies, London.

Rose, R. (1975) Overloaded government: the problem outlined, *European Studies Newsletter*, 5, 13-18.

Rousseau, Mme (1997) rapporteur on 'Extrait des débats à l'Assemblée Nationale, *Les Dossiers de l'ADEPHA*, Association des Directeurs d'Etablissements d'Hébergement pour Personnes Agées (ADEPHA), January, Paris, pp.6-7.

Saunders, R. (1990) Transfrontier migration of French elderly people into Belgian residential care, PSSRU Discussion Paper 735, University of Kent, Canterbury.

Schauffler, H.H., Howland, J. and Cobb, J. (1992) Using chronic disease risk factors to adjust Medicare capitation payments, *Health Care Financing Review*, Fall, 14, 1, 79-90.

Schopflin, P. (1991) Dépendance et solidarités mieux aider les personnes âgées, Paris.
Shanas, E. (1979) Social myth as hypothesis: the case of the family relations of old people, *The Gerontologist*, 19, 3-9.
Shanas, E., Townsend, P., Wedderburn, D., Friis, H., Milhoj, P. and Stehouwer, J. (1968) *Old People in Three Industrial Societies*, Routledge and Kegan Paul, London.
Simon, M.-O. (1997) Prestation dépendance: les bénéficiaires satisfaits des expérimentations réalisées en 1995 et en 1996, *Crédoc: Consommation et Modes de Vie*, Centre de Recherche pour l'Etude et l'Observation des Conditions de Vie, Paris.
Social Services Inspectorate (1987) *From Home Help to Home Care: An Analysis of Policy, Resourcing and Service Management*, Social Services Inspectorate, Department of Health, London.
Social Services Inspectorate (1988) *Managing to Care: A Study of First Line Managers in Social Services Departments in Day and Domiciliary Care*, Social Services Inspectorate, Department of Health, London.
Soubie, R., Portos, J.-L. and Prieur, C. (1994) *Livre blanc sur le système de santé et d'assurance maladie*, Commissariat général du plan, La Documentation Française, Paris.
Spector, W.O. and Kemper, P. (1994) Disability and cognitive impairment criteria: targeting those who need the most home care, *The Gerontologist*, 34, 640-51.
Stewart, J.D. (1986) *The New Management of Local Government*, Allen and Unwin, London.
Tennstedt, S., Crawford, S. and McKinlay, J. (1993) Is family care on the decline? A longitudinal investigation of the substitution of formal long-term care services for informal care, *The Millbank Quarterly*, 71, 601-24.
Titmuss, R. (1968) *Commitment to Welfare*, Allen and Unwin, London.
Townsend, P. (1962) *The Last Refuge*, Routledge and Kegan Paul, London.
Wan, T.T.H. and Weissert, W. (1981) Social support networks, patient status and institutionalisation, *Research on Aging*, 3, 2, 240-56.
Warburton, R.W. (1994) *Home and Away*, Department of Health, HMSO, London.
White Paper (1983) *Financial Management in Government Departments*, Cmnd 9058, HMSO, London.

White Paper (1989) *Caring for People: Community Care in the Next Decade and Beyond*, Cm 849, HMSO, London.

White Paper (1996) *A New Partnership for Care in Old Age*, Cm 3242, HMSO, London.

White Paper (1997) *Financing Care Partnerships*, Cm 3563, HMSO, London.

Wistow, G., Knapp, M.R., Hardy, B. and Allen, C. (1994) *Social Care in a Mixed Economy*, Open University Press, Buckingham.

Wistow, G., Knapp, M.R., Hardy, B., Forder, J. and Kendall, J. (1996) *Social Care Markets: Progress and Prospects*, Open University Press, Buckingham.

Young, M. and Willmott, P. (1957) *Family and Kinship in East London*, Routledge and Kegan Paul, London.

Subject index

Author index